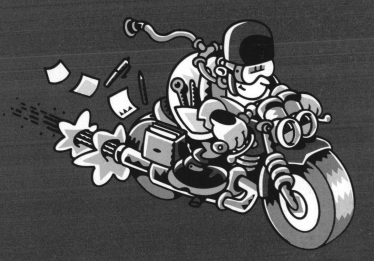

Cardiology

Series editor
Wilfred Yeo
BMedSci, MB, ChB, MD, MRCP
Senior Lecturer in Medicine,
Medicine/Clinical
Pharmacology and
Therapeutics,
University of
Sheffield

Faculty advisor
Mark Noble
DSc, MD, PhD, FRCP, FESC
Weston Professor of
Cardiovascular Medicine,
National Heart and Lung
Institute,
Imperial College of
Science, Technology, and
Medicine, and
Charing Cross Hospital,
London

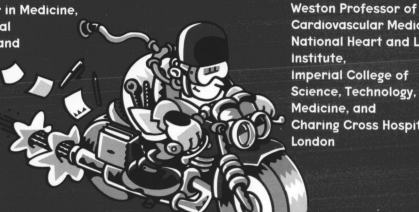

Cardiology

Anjana Siva
MA, BChir, MRCP
Research Registrar
Department of Clinical
Pharmacology,
Addenbrooke's Hospital,
Cambridge

Mark Noble
DSc, MD, PhD, FRCP, FESC
Weston Professor of
Cardiovascular Medicine,
National Heart and Lung
Institute,
Imperial College of Science,
Technology, and Medicine,
and
Charing Cross Hospital,
London

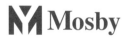 Mosby

London Edinburgh New York Philadelphia Sydney Toronto

Editor	Louise Crowe
Development Editor	Linda Horrell
Project Manager	Lindy van den Berghe
Designer	Greg Smith
Layout	Kate Walshaw
Illustration Management	Mick Ruddy
Illustrator	Jenni Miller
Cover Design	Greg Smith
Index	Janine Ross

ISBN 0 7234 3152 3

Copyright © Harcourt Publishers Limited 1999.

Published in 1999 by Mosby, an imprint of Harcourt Publishers Limited.

Text set in Crash Course—VAG Light; captions in Crash Course—VAG Thin.

Cataloguing in Publication Data
Catalogue records for this book are available from the British Library and the US Library of Congress.

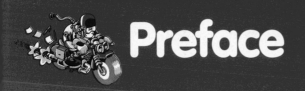

Preface

Cardiology is a varied and exciting field comprising a wide range of acute and chronic disorders. No final year medical student can avoid learning the basics of cardiology because the speciality is well represented in all aspects of the final examination, and rightly so because the more common cardiac conditions such as ischaemic heart disease, cardiac failure, and valve disease are frequently seen in practice by all junior doctors.

This book is designed to cover all aspects of cardiac disease and its management. The management of acute emergencies is laid out clearly in the form of flow charts. Clinical trials have been mentioned wherever relevant to enable students to see the effect of the results of these trials on medical practice.

Care has been taken to present diseases in an interesting and concise manner with management plans that are up to date and particularly relevant for final year students and junior doctors. Emphasis has been placed upon the importance of good history taking and examination skills and the need to approach all problems in a logical manner.

I hope you find this text a useful revision tool. Good luck!

Anjana Siva

Over the past 30 years it has been my privilege to enjoy rapport with many generations of medical students. In recent years this has involved a revolution in teaching methods and a new curriculum. Students are being introduced to clinical cardiology from the beginning of their studies.

Although designed as a revision course, this book contains all the student needs to know about cardiology for MB finals. It is based on clinical experience. In the new system of learning the student should explore, from this clinical knowledge, the underlying anatomy and physiology. Then it is possible to understand why the clinical features are as they are from logical reasoning from first principles. The companion book – *Crash Course Cardiovascular System* – is recommended to aid this process of deeper understanding.

Beware, however, of the danger of learning primarily specialties and systems. The patient must be understood as a whole person.

Mark Noble

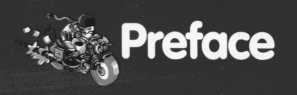

Preface

So you have an exam in medicine and you don't know where to start? The answer is easy—start with *Crash Course*. Medicine is fun to learn if you can bring it to life with patients who need their problems solving. Conventional medical textbooks are written back-to-front, starting with the diagnosis and then describing the disease. This is because medicine evolved by careful observations and descriptions of individual diseases for which, until this century, there was no treatment. Modern medicine is about problem solving, learning methods to find the right path through the differential diagnosis, and offering treatment promptly.

This series of books has been designed to help you solve common medical problems by starting with the patient and extracting the salient points in the history, examination, and investigations. Part II gives you essential information on the physical examination and investigations as seen through the eyes of practising doctors in their specialty. Once the diagnosis is made, you can refer to Part III to confirm that the diagnosis is correct and get advice regarding treatment.

Throughout the series we have included informative diagrams and hints and tips boxes to simplify your learning. The books are meant as revision tools, but are comprehensive, accurate, and well balanced and should enable you to learn each subject well. To check that you did learn something from the book (rather than just flashing it in front of your eyes!), we have added a self-assessment section in the usual format of most medical exams—multiple-choice and short-answer questions (with answers), and patient management problems for self-directed learning. Good luck!

Wilf Yeo
Series Editor (Clinical)

Contents

Contents

Contents

To my mother and father   AS

Acknowledgements

I would like to thank the following individuals for their help in providing material for this text:
Miss S Bland for providing the exercise ECG.
Mr D Cuthbert for providing information on cholesterol lowering trials.
Miss A Hall for providing the ECG showing atrial flutter.
Dr MO Sullivan for providing the ECG showing left ventricular hypertrophy.
Dr S Haydock for providing the retinal photos.

Anjana Siva

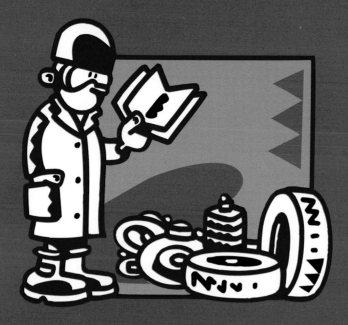

THE PATIENT PRESENTS WITH

1. Chest Pain

DIFFERENTIAL DIAGNOSIS OF CHEST PAIN

Chest pain is one of the most common presenting complaints seen by cardiologists. It is important to remember that:
- There are many causes of chest pain.
- Some are life-threatening and require prompt diagnosis and treatment whereas others are more benign.

The first differentiation to be made is between cardiac and non-cardiac chest pain (Fig. 1.1)

HISTORY TO FOCUS ON THE DIFFERENTIAL DIAGNOSIS OF CHEST PAIN

Because the differential diagnosis is so diverse a thorough history is very important.

Presenting complaint
Differentiation depends upon a detailed history of the pain with particular emphasis on the following characteristics of the pain (Fig. 1.2):
- Continuous or intermittent.
- Duration.
- Position of the pain—central or lateral/posterior.
- Exacerbating factors—exertion, emotion, food, posture, movement, breathing.
- Radiation of the pain—to neck, arms, head.
- Quality of pain—crushing, burning, stabbing.

Past medical history
This may provide important clues:
- A history of ischaemic heart disease.
- A history of peptic ulcer disease or of frequent ingestion of non-steroidal anti-inflammatory drugs.

Differential diagnosis of chest pain	
System involved	**Pathology**
cardiac	myocardial infarction angina pectoris pericarditis prolapse of the mitral valve
vascular	aortic dissection
respiratory (all tend to give rise to pleuritic pain)	pulmonary embolus pneumonia pneumothorax pulmonary neoplasm
gastrointestinal	oesophagitis due to gastric reflux oesophageal tear peptic ulcer biliary disease
musculoskeletal	cervical nerve root compression by cervical disc costochondritis fractured rib
neurological	herpes zoster

Fig. 1.1 Differential diagnosis of chest pain.

- Recent operations—cardiothoracic surgery may be complicated by Dressler's syndrome, mediastinitis, ischaemic heart disease or pulmonary embolus (PE).
- Pericarditis may be preceded by a prodromal viral illness.
- Pulmonary embolus may be preceded by a period of inactivity (e.g. a recent operation, illness, or long journey).
- Hypertension is a risk factor for both ischaemic heart disease and dissection of the thoracic aorta.

Drug history, family history, and social history
Other risk factors for ischaemic heart disease such as a positive family history and smoking should be excluded.

A history of heavy alcohol intake is a risk factor for gastritis and peptic ulcer disease.

Characteristics of different types of chest pain					
Characteristic	Myocardial ischaemia	Pericarditis	Pleuritic pain	Gastrointestinal disease	Musculoskeletal
Quality of pain	crushing, tight or bandlike	sharp (may be crushing)	sharp	burning	usually sharp may be a dull ache
Site of pain	central anterior chest	central anterior	anywhere (usually very localized pain)	central	may be anywhere
Radiation	to throat, jaw or arms	usually no radiation	usually no radiation	to throat	to arms or around chest to back
Exacerbating and relieving factors	exacerbated by exertion, anxiety, cold; relieved by rest and by glyceryl trinitrate	exacerbated when lying back relieved by sitting forward	exacerbated by breathing, coughing, or moving; relieved when stop breathing	peptic ulcer pain often relieved by food and antacids (cholecystitis and oesophageal pain are exacerbated by food)	may be exacerbated by pressing on chest wall or moving neck
Associated features	patient often sweaty, breathless, and shocked; may feel nauseated	fever, recent viral illness (e.g. rash, arthralgia)	cough, haemoptysis, breathlessness; shock with pulmonary embolus	excessive wind	other affected joints; patient otherwise looks very well

Fig. 1.2 Characteristics of different types of chest pain.

When a patient presents as a hospital emergency with cardiac chest pain, try to differentiate diagnoses for which thrombolysis is contraindicated from those for which it is indicated. Thrombolysis is contraindicated in pericarditis and dissection of the thoracic aorta.

EXAMINATION OF PATIENTS WHO HAVE CHEST PAIN

Points to note on examination of the patient who has chest pain are shown in Fig. 1.3.

Inspection

On inspection, look for:
- Signs of shock (e.g. pallor, sweating)—may indicate myocardial infarction (MI), dissecting aorta, PE.
- Laboured breathing—may indicate MI leading to left ventricular failure (LVF) or a pulmonary cause.

- Signs of vomiting—suggests MI or an oesophageal cause.
- Coughing—suggests LVF, pneumonia.

Cardiovascular system

Note the following:
- Pulse and blood pressure—any abnormal rhythm, tachycardia, bradycardia, hypotension, hypertension? Inequalities in the pulses or blood pressure between different extremities are seen in aortic dissection.
- Mucous membranes—pallor could suggest angina due to anaemia; cyanosis suggests hypoxia.
- Any increase in jugular venous pressure—a sign of right ventricular infarction or pulmonary embolus.
- Carotid pulse waveform—a collapsing pulse is seen with aortic regurgitation, which can complicate aortic dissection. It is slow rising if angina is due to aortic stenosis.
- Displaced apex beat, abnormal cardiac impulses (e.g. paradoxical movement in anterior myocardial infarction).
- On auscultation—listen for a pericardial rub, third heart sound (a feature of LVF), mitral or aortic regurgitation (features of myocardial infarction or dissection respectively), aortic stenosis (causes angina).

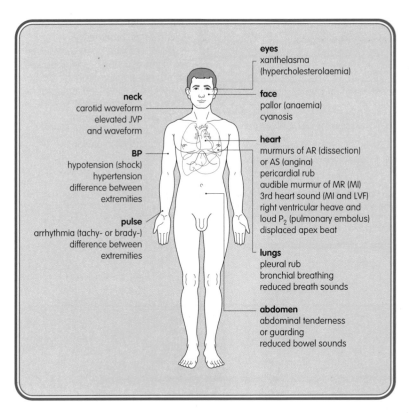

neck
carotid waveform
elevated JVP
and waveform

BP
hypotension (shock)
hypertension
difference between
extremities

pulse
arrhythmia (tachy- or brady-)
difference between
extremities

eyes
xanthelasma
(hypercholesterolaemia)

face
pallor (anaemia)
cyanosis

heart
murmurs of AR (dissection)
or AS (angina)
pericardial rub
audible murmur of MR (MI)
3rd heart sound (MI and LVF)
right ventricular heave and
loud P_2 (pulmonary embolus)
displaced apex beat

lungs
pleural rub
bronchial breathing
reduced breath sounds

abdomen
abdominal tenderness
or guarding
reduced bowel sounds

Fig. 1.3 Points to note when examining a patient who has chest pain. (AR, aortic regurgitation; AS, aortic stenosis; BP, blood pressure; JVP, jugular venous pressure; LVF, left ventricular failure; MI, myocardial infarction; MR, mitral regurgitation; P_2, pulmonary component of the second heart sound.)

Respiratory system

Note the following signs:

- Breathlessness or cyanosis.
- Unequal hemithorax expansion
  —a sign of pneumonia and pneumothorax.
- Abnormal dullness over lung fields
  —a sign of pneumonia.
- Any bronchial breathing or pleural rub
  —signs of pneumonia and pleurisy.

Gastrointestinal system

Specifically look for:

- Abdominal tenderness or guarding.
- Scanty or absent bowel sounds—suggests an ileus (e.g. due to perforated peptic ulcer and peritonitis).

INVESTIGATION OF PATIENTS WHO HAVE CHEST PAIN

A summary of tests used to investigate chest pain is shown in Fig. 1.4 and an algorithm is shown in Fig. 1.5.

Blood tests

These include:

- Cardiac enzymes—may be elevated in MI from 4 hours after the onset of infarction.
- Full blood count—anaemia may exacerbate angina.
- Renal function and electrolytes—may be abnormal if the patient has been vomiting, leading to dehydration and hypokalaemia, or due to diuretic therapy.
- Arterial blood gases—hypoxia is a sign of PE and LVF, hypocapnoea is seen with hyperventilation.
- Liver function tests and serum amylase—deranged in cholecystitis and peptic ulcer disease.

Electrocardiography

Findings may include:

- Bundle branch block (BBB)—if new this may be due to MI; if it is old MI cannot be diagnosed from the ECG.
- ST elevation in absence of BBB indicates acute MI (rarely it is due to Prinzmetal's angina).
- Fully developed Q waves—indicate old MI (i.e. over 24 hours old).
- Atrial fibrillation secondary to any pulmonary disease or ischaemia.

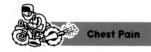

First-line tests to exclude a chest pain emergency	
Test	**Diagnosis**
arterial blood gases	in the dyspnoeic patient severe hypoxaemia suggests pulmonary embolus, LVF or pneumonia
cardiac enzymes	may be normal in first 4 hours after MI, but CK-MB will then increase
ECG	if normal excludes MI, although evidence for this may emerge upon observation
CXR	widened mediastinum suggests aortic dissection; may show pleural effusion or pulmonary consolidation
CT scan	carry out urgently for suspected aortic dissection

Fig. 1.4 First-line tests to exclude a chest pain emergency. (CK-MB, creatine kinase composed of M (muscle) and B (brain) subunits, which is found primarily in cardiac muscle; CT, computed tomography; CXR, chest radiography; ECG, electrocardiography; LVF, left ventricular failure; MI, myocardial infarction.)

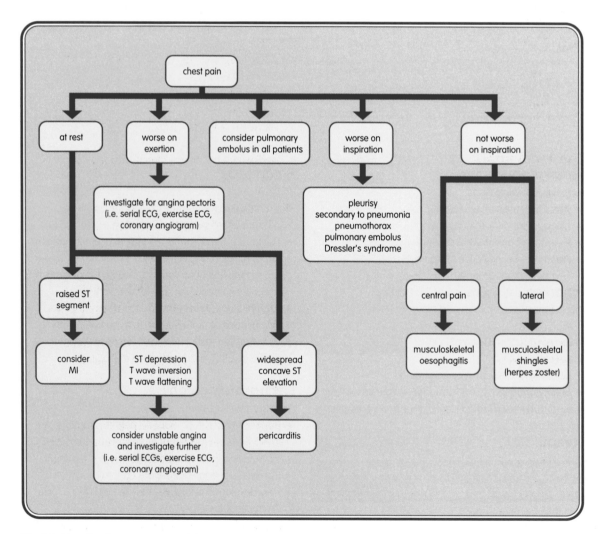

Fig. 1.5 Algorithm for investigation of chest pain. (MI, myocardial infarction; UA, unstable angina.)

- ST depression in absence of BBB—indicates myocardial ischaemia. At rest this equates with unstable angina or non-Q wave infarction; on exertion this equates with effort-induced angina pectoris or tachyarrhythmias.

In the event of a large PE the classical changes to be seen are:
- Sinus tachycardia (or atrial fibrillation).
- Tall P waves in lead II (right atrial dilatation).
- Right axis deviation and right bundle branch block.
- S wave in lead I, Q wave in lead III, and inverted T wave in lead III (SI QIII TIII pattern seen only with very large PE).

Acute MI is diagnosed from the history of chest pain and raised ST segments or new left BBB. Consider PE in every case, and if strongly suspected treat as PE until a ventilation perfusion scan can be performed.

Chest radiograph
The following signs may be seen:
- Cardiomegaly.
- Widening of the mediastinum in aortic dissection.
- Lung lesions.
- Pleural and pericardial effusions.
- Oligaemic lung fields in PE.

Echocardiography
This may reveal:
- Pericardial effusion—suggests pericarditis or dissection.
- Regional myocardial dysfunction—a feature of myocardial infarction or ischaemia.
- Aortic dissection with false lumen.
- Aortic or mitral valve abnormalities.

Computed tomography scanning and magnetic resonance imaging
These are the most sensitive methods for excluding aortic dissection and should be performed urgently if this diagnosis is suspected.

It is sometimes possible to visualize PE with spiral computed tomography (CT) scanning.

Ventilation/perfusion (V/Q) scan
This excludes PE in most cases if performed promptly. If the scan is negative and PE is strongly suspected a more sensitive test is a pulmonary angiogram.

Exercise tolerance test or myocardial perfusion scan
This may be performed at a later date if angina is suspected.

CENTRAL CHEST PAIN AT REST OF RECENT ONSET IN AN ILL PATIENT

The importance of this subject is that this situation represents a medical emergency requiring rapid diagnosis and treatment.

It is necessary in this situation to distinguish between:
- MI (see Chapter 14).
- Unstable angina.
- Pericarditis.
- Dissection of thoracic aorta.
- PE.
- Mediastinitis secondary to oesophageal tear.
- Non-cardiac chest pain.

Thrombolysis
This is the treatment for MI with an onset less than 24 hours previously. The pain of MI is characteristically a tight crushing band-like pain that may radiate to the jaws or arms.

Conditions for which thrombolysis is contraindicated
The following guidelines help differentiate MI from disorders in which thrombolysis can be lethal.

Pericarditis
In pericarditis:
- The patient may have a prodromal viral illness.
- Pain may be exacerbated by breathing movements.
- There may be concomitant indications of infection.

Examination may reveal a pericardial rub—an added sound (or sounds) in the cardiac area on auscultation, which has a scratchy quality and seems close to the ears.

If complicated by pericardial effusion, there may be:
- An impalpable cardiac impulse.
- An increased cardiothoracic ratio on the chest radiograph, with a globular shaped heart shadow.

The ECG shows characteristic concave-upwards raised ST segments in all leads except AVR. Thrombolysis is contraindicated because it causes haemopericardium.

Dissection of the thoracic aorta

The pain is sharp and tearing. There is often radiation of the pain to the back. There may be a previous history of or current hypertension.

On examination, the patient may be shocked, and there may be delays between the major pulses (e.g. right brachial vs left brachial, brachial vs femoral).

Chest radiography may show a widened mediastinum. The ECG will not show ST elevation unless the coronary ostia are dissected. Confirmation may require high-resolution spiral CT scanning, echocardiography, or magnetic resonance imaging (which is the best investigation when available; Fig. 1.6).

Thrombolysis is contraindicated because it causes massive bleeding from the aorta.

Overview of dissection of the thoracic aorta	
predisposing factors	hypertension bicuspid aortic valve pregnancy Marfan, Turner's, Noonan's syndrome connective tissue diseases—SLE, Ehlers–Danlos syndrome men > women middle age
pathophysiology	damage to the media and high intraluminal pressure causing an intimal tear blood enters and dissects the luminal plane of the media creating a false lumen
classification	Stanford classification: type A—all dissections involving the ascending aorta; type B—all dissections not involving the ascending aorta
symptoms	central tearing chest pain radiating to the back further complications as the dissection involves branches of the aorta: coronary ostia—myocardial infarction; carotid or spinal arteries—hemiplegia, dysphasia, or paraplegia; mesenteric arteries—abdominal pain
signs	shocked, cyanosed, sweating blood pressure and pulses differ between extremities aortic regurgitation cardiac tamponade cardiac failure
investigation	CXR—widened mediastinum +/– fluid in costophrenic angle ECG—may be ST elevation CT/MRI—best investigations, show aortic false lumen transoesophageal echo if available also very sensitive echocardiography—may show pericardial effusion if dissection extends proximally; tamponade may occur
management	pain relief—diamorphine intravenous access—central and arterial line fluid replacement—initially colloid then blood when available —crossmatch at least 10 units blood pressure control—intravenous nitroprusside infusion or labetalol infusion if no cardiac failure—keep blood pressure < 120/80 mmHg surgery for all type A dissections medical management and possibly surgery for type B

Fig. 1.6 Overview of dissection of the thoracic aorta. (CT, computed tomography; CXR, chest radiography; ECG, electrocardiography; MRI, magnetic resonance imaging.)

Mediastinitis

This is unusual and need not usually be considered unless there is a possibility of an oesophageal leak (e.g. after endoscopy or oesophageal surgery).

Pulmonary embolus

Pulmonary emboli may present as acute chest pain in an ill patient or as intermittent chest pain in a relatively well patient. For this reason it is crucial to suspect PE in all patients who have chest pain that is not typically anginal.

The pain of a PE may be pleuritic or tight in nature and may be located anywhere in the chest. It may be accompanied by the following symptoms and signs:

- Dyspnoea.
- Dry cough or haemoptysis.
- Hypotension and sweating.
- Sudden collapse with syncope.

Massive PE will cause collapse with cardiac arrest. The ECG may show ventricular tachyarrhythmias or sinus rhythm with electromechanical dissociation.

Patients will often experience a sense of 'impending doom' or profound anxiety.

Conditions predisposing to clot formation in the deep veins of the leg are associated with a high incidence of PE (Fig. 1.7).

Conditions predisposing to deep venous thrombosis	
Condition	**Examples**
immobility	prolonged bed rest for any reason, long air journeys
postoperative	abdominal and pelvic surgery, leg and hip surgery
haemoconcentration	diuretic therapy, polycythaemia
hypercoagulable states	malignancy, oral contraceptive pill, protein C/protein S deficiency, etc.
venous stasis (poor flow of venous blood)	congestive cardiac failure, atrial fibrillation (formation of thrombus in the right ventricle may result in PE)

Fig. 1.7 Conditions predisposing to deep venous thrombosis.

The mortality rate resulting from PE is approximately 10% so appropriate investigations to exclude PE should be carried out promptly and anticoagulation commenced using either intravenous heparin as an infusion or an appropriate low-molecular weight heparin preparation subcutaneously. If PE is confirmed warfarin therapy should be commenced.

2. Dyspnoea

Dyspnoea is an uncomfortable awareness of one's own breathing. It is considered abnormal only when it occurs at a level of physical activity not normally expected to cause any problem.

DIFFERENTIAL DIAGNOSIS OF DYSPNOEA

Dyspnoea is the main symptom of many cardiac and pulmonary diseases. A working knowledge of the differential diagnosis is required to be able to differentiate acute life-threatening conditions from those that do not require immediate treatment (Fig 2.1).

HISTORY TO FOCUS ON THE DIFFERENTIAL DIAGNOSIS OF DYSPNOEA

Differentiation depends upon a detailed history of the dyspnoea (Fig. 2.2) with particular emphasis on the following details:

- Acute or chronic.
- Continuous or intermittent.
- Exacerbating and relieving factors—such as exertion, lying flat (suggests orthopnoea in pulmonary oedema), sleep (suggests paroxysmal nocturnal dyspnoea, PND, which is waking from sleep gasping for breath in left ventricular failure (LVF).
- Associated features such as cough—ask for details of sputum production—yellow–green sputum suggests pneumonia or exacerbation of chronic obstructive airways disease (COAD); pink frothy sputum suggests LVF; haemoptysis can be a feature of pneumonia, pulmonary embolus (PE), and carcinoma of the lung.
- Chest pain—ask for details of location, nature of pain, radiation, etc. (see Chapter 1).
- Palpitations—ask about rate and rhythm.
- Ankle oedema—suggestive of congestive cardiac failure, swelling usually worse at the end of the day and best first thing in the morning.
- Wheeze—suggestive of airways obstruction (i.e. asthma, COAD, or neoplasm of the lung causing airway obstruction). Wheeze can also occur during LVF.

Fig. 2.1 Differential diagnosis of dyspnoea. (COAD, chronic obstructive airways disease.)

Differential diagnosis of dyspnoea	
System involved	Pathology
cardiac	cardiac failure coronary artery disease valvular heart disease—aortic stenosis, aortic regurgitation, mitral stenosis/regurgitation, pulmonary stenosis cardiac arrhythmias
respiratory	pulmonary embolus airway obstruction—COAD, asthma pneumothorax pulmonary parenchymal disease (e.g. pneumonia, pulmonary fibrosis, lung neoplasm) pleural effusion chest wall limitation—myopathy, neuropathy (e.g. Guillain–Barré disease), rib fracture, kyphoscoliosis
other	obesity limiting chest wall movement anaemia psychogenic hyperventilation acidosis (e.g. aspirin overdose, diabetic ketoacidosis)

	Cardiac failure	Coronary artery disease	Pulmonary embolus	Pneumothorax	COAD and asthma

Presenting history for different diseases causing dyspnoea

	Cardiac failure	Coronary artery disease	Pulmonary embolus	Pneumothorax	COAD and asthma
Acute or chronic	may be acute or chronic	acute	acute (less commonly recurrent small PEs may present as chronic dyspnoea)	acute	acute or chronic
Continuous or intermittent	may be continuous or intermittent	usually intermittent, but an acute MI may lead to continuous and severe LVF	continuous	continuous	continuous or intermittent; these disorders range from the acute, life-threatening exacerbations to chronic relatively mild episodes
Exacerbating and relieving factors	exacerbated by exertion and lying flat (orthopnoea and PND may occur) and occasionally food; relieved by rest, sitting up, oxygen, and GTN	exacerbated by exertion, cold; may be relieved by oxygen			exacerbated by exertion, pulmonary infections, allergens (e.g. pollen, animal danders); relieved by bronchodilator inhalers
Associated features	may be chest pain (ischaemia may cause LVF); palpitations—arrhythmias may precipitate LVF; cough with pink frothy sputum	chest pain (central crushing pain radiating to the left arm or throat) and sweating; occasionally palpitations—atrial fibrillation may be precipitated by ischaemia	pleuritic chest pain (sharp, localized pain worse on breathing and coughing) and bright red haemoptysis; atrial fibrillation may occur	pleuritic chest pain there may be a history of chest trauma	cough with sputum; pleuritic chest pain if associated infection; wheeze

Fig. 2.2 Presenting history for different diseases causing dyspnoea. (COAD, chronic obstructive airways disease; GTN, glyceryl trinitrate; LVF, left ventricular failure; MI, myocardial infarction; PE, pulmonary embolus; PND, paroxysmal nocturnal dyspnoea.)

EXAMINATION OF DYSPNOEIC PATIENTS

As usual a thorough examination will be needed because the differential diagnosis is potentially wide (Fig. 2.3).

Inspection
Note the following:
- Pyrexia—suggests infection (PE or myocardial infarction may be associated with a low-grade pyrexia).
- Signs of shock—pallor, sweating—suggests acute LVF, pneumonia, PE.
- Inspect for laboured or obstructed breathing (any intercostal recession?), tachypnoea, or cyanosis. One or more usually present with resting dyspnoea.
- Cough—suggests acute LVF, pneumonia; note the appearance of the sputum (always ask to look in the sputum pot if it is present).

- Appearance of hands and fingers—such as clubbing, carbon dioxide retention flap.
- Appearance of chest—a barrel-shaped chest is a feature of emphysema, kyphoscoliosis causes distortion.

Cardiovascular system
Check the following:
- Pulse and blood pressure—any abnormal rhythm, tachycardia, bradycardia, hypotension, hypertension?
- Mucous membranes—pallor suggests dyspnoea in anaemia; cyanosis suggests hypoxia in LVF, COAD, PE, pneumonia, and lung collapse.
- Carotid pulse waveform and jugular venous pressure (JVP)—JVP is elevated in cardiac failure and conditions causing pulmonary hypertension (e.g. PE, COAD).
- Apex beat—displacement suggests cardiac enlargement, and a right ventricular heave suggests pulmonary hypertension.

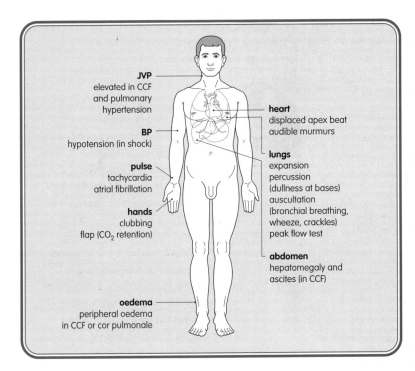

JVP
elevated in CCF
and pulmonary
hypertension

BP
hypotension (in shock)

pulse
tachycardia
atrial fibrillation

hands
clubbing
flap (CO$_2$ retention)

oedema
peripheral oedema
in CCF or cor pulmonale

heart
displaced apex beat
audible murmurs

lungs
expansion
percussion
(dullness at bases)
auscultation
(bronchial breathing,
wheeze, crackles)
peak flow test

abdomen
hepatomegaly and
ascites (in CCF)

Fig. 2.3 Points to note when examining a dyspnoeic patient. (BP, blood pressure; CCF, congestive cardiac failure; JVP, jugular venous pressure.)

- Heart sounds—note any audible murmurs or added heart sounds—third heart sound in LVF; mitral regurgitation or aortic valve lesions may cause LVF).
- Peripheral oedema.

Respiratory system

Check the following:
- Expansion—unequal thorax expansion is a sign of pneumonia or pneumothorax.
- Vocal fremitus—enhanced vocal fremitus is a sign of consolidation; reduced vocal fremitus is a sign of effusion and pneumothorax.
- Abnormal dullness over hemithorax with reduced expansion—suggests pneumonia.
- Stony dullness at one or both lung bases—suggests pleural effusion.
- Hyperresonance over hemithorax with less expansion— suggests pneumothorax.
- Bilateral hyperresonance with loss of cardiac dullness—suggests emphysema.
- Bronchial breathing—suggests pneumonia; or crepitations—suggests pneumonia, pulmonary oedema, pulmonary fibrosis.
- Wheeze—asthma, COAD, cardiac asthma in LVF.
- Peak flow test—this is part of every examination of the respiratory system and you should always ask to

do this. Explain the technique to the patient clearly and then perform three attempts and take the best out of three. Peak flow will be reduced in active asthma and COAD.

Gastrointestinal system
Examine for hepatomegaly and ascites—seen in congestive cardiac failure or isolated right-sided failure.

INVESTIGATION OF DYSPNOEIC PATIENTS

A summary of first-line tests to exclude emergencies is shown in Fig. 2.4.

Blood tests
These include:
- Full blood count—may reveal anaemia or leucocytosis (in pneumonia).
- Urea and electrolytes—deranged due to diuretic treatment of cardiac failure, possible syndrome of inappropriate antidiuretic hormone secretion in pneumonia.
- Cardiac enzymes—elevated if dyspnoea secondary to myocardial infarction.

13

First-line tests to exclude a dyspnoeic emergency	
Test	**Diagnosis**
CXR	acute LVF—pulmonary oedema +/– large heart shadow acute asthma—clear overexpanded lungs pneumothorax—absence of lung markings between lung edge and chest wall pneumonia—consolidation.
ECG	look for evidence of MI, ischaemia, pulmonary embolus
arterial blood gases	normal pH excludes uncompensated acute hyperventilation or respiratory failure; hypoxia suggests LVF or significant lung disease (use the level of hypoxia to guide the need for oxygen therapy or artificial ventilation)
peak flow	reduced in airway obstruction (asthma, COAD), but may also be reduced in sick patients because of weakness (it is an effort-dependent test)

Fig. 2.4 First-line tests to exclude a dyspnoeic emergency. (COAD, chronic obstructive airways disease; CXR, chest radiography; ECG, electrocardiography; LVF, left ventricular failure; MI, myocardial infarction.)

Arterial blood gas results in dyspnoeic patients			
	pO$_2$ (kPa)	pCO$_2$ (kPa)	pH
Normal range	10.5–13.5	5.0–6.0	7.36–7.44
Ventilatory failure (e.g. chronic obstructive airways disease, severe asthma with exhaustion)	7.0	9.0	7.30
Acute hyperventilation	13.0	4.0	7.48
Hypoxia (e.g. left ventricular failure, pulmonary embolus)	7.5	4.0	7.41

Fig. 2.5 Examples of arterial blood gas results in dyspnoeic patients. The low pH in ventilatory failure is secondary to an acute retention of carbon dioxide. The high pH in acute hyperventilation results from an acute loss of carbon dioxide (respiratory alkalosis). The case of hypoxia shown here has led to hyperventilation and a fall of carbon dioxide and must have been present for some time because the pH is compensated to normal by renal excretion of bicarbonate.

- Liver function tests—deranged in hepatic congestion secondary to congestive cardiac failure.
- Arterial blood gases (Fig. 2.5).

Notes on blood gases:
- Hypoxia and hypocapnoea are seen in LVF and pulmonary embolus (this shows a drop in pCO$_2$ due to hyperventilation as a response to hypoxia).
- Hypoxia and hypercapnoea may occur in COAD and severe asthma —in the former condition this is because the respiratory centre has readjusted to the chronic hypoxia and oxygen therapy causes the blood pO$_2$ to rise and the respiratory drive to fall, so ventilation is reduced and the blood pCO$_2$ rises. In asthma, exhaustion causes the ventilatory drive to fall off and the pCO$_2$ to rise, this precedes respiratory arrest and is an indication for artificial ventilation of the patient).
- Arterial pH—in acute conditions such as acute LVF, pulmonary embolus, pneumothorax, and early asthma a respiratory alkalosis occurs (i.e. a low pCO$_2$ and a high pH >7.4). The kidneys have not yet compensated by excreting bicarbonate.
- In COAD with chronic CO$_2$ retention the pH is normal as metabolic compensation has occurred and bicarbonate levels rise due to renal retention of bicarbonate (this takes a few days to occur).
- In severe asthma with acute CO$_2$ retention the pH falls as the pCO$_2$ rises as there has been insufficient time for metabolic compensation to occur.

Electrocardiography

This may show:

- Ischaemic changes may be seen in patients with coronary artery disease.
- Sinus tachycardia with SI, QIII, TIII (see p. 7) in patients who have had a large PE.
- Atrial fibrillation—may be seen secondary to any lung pathology or ischaemia.

Chest radiography

Note the following:

- Cardiomegaly in cardiac failure. Pulmonary oedema may also be seen.
- Focal lung consolidation in pneumonia (shadowing of a lung segment with an air bronchogram).
- Pleural effusion—suggests PE, infection, or cardiac failure.
- Hyperexpanded lung fields in emphysema (ability to count more than six rib spaces over the lung fields); bullae may be seen in emphysema.
- Presence of a pneumothorax—ask for a film in full expiration if this is suspected.
- Oligaemic lung fields in PE.

Echocardiography

This may reveal:

- Left ventricular failure.
- Valve lesions.
- Left atrial myxoma.
- Right ventricular hypertrophy and pulmonary hypertension.

Ventilation/perfusion scan

This may be used to exclude PE—a mismatched defect with good ventilation and no perfusion is diagnostic of a PE; matched defects are due to infection or COAD or pulmonary scar tissue.

If this is negative or equivocal in a high-risk patient it would be reasonable to proceed to pulmonary angiography. This is the most sensitive test for a PE.

Computed tomography scanning

This is used to obtain detailed visualization of pulmonary fibrosis or small peripheral tumours that cannot be reached with a bronchoscope.

Pulmonary function tests

These tests are used to investigate:

- Lung volumes—increased in COAD, reduced in restrictive lung disease.
- Flow volume loop—scalloped in COAD.
- Carbon monoxide transfer—reduced in the presence of normal airway function in restrictive lung diseases.

Notes on dyspnoea and arterial blood gases:
- **The life-threatening cardiopulmonary conditions, respiratory failure and carbon monoxide poisoning, may not cause prominent dyspnoea, but may present as coma or semi-coma.**
- **Severe hypoxia or tissue underperfusion causes metabolic acidosis (low pH with normal or low pCO_2.**
- **Most importantly—arterial blood gases must be performed for all dyspnoeic patients at presentation.**

DYSPNOEA AT REST OF RECENT ONSET IN AN ILL PATIENT

The importance of this subject is that this situation represents a cardiopulmonary emergency requiring rapid diagnosis and treatment.

It is necessary in this situation to distinguish between the life-threatening causes:

- Acute LVF.
- Life-threatening asthma.
- PE.
- Tension pneumothorax.
- Fulminant pneumonia.

Pneumothorax

Pneumothorax (or air in the pleural space) may cause acute or chronic dyspnoea. There are a number of possible causes, all creating a connection between the pleural space and the atmosphere (either via the chest wall or the airways). These include:

- Trauma (e.g. a blow to the chest resulting in fracture of the ribs or insertion of a central venous cannula).
- Rupture of bullae on the surface of the lung—this occurs in some otherwise healthy young patients (more commonly in men than in women) or in patients who have emphysema.

Tension pneumothorax can occur if the air continues to accumulate in the pleural cavity resulting in a progressive increase in pressure and displacement of the mediastinum away from the side of the lesion. This is characterized by the following clinical signs:

- Severe and worsening dyspnoea.
- Displaced trachea and apex beat.
- Hyper-resonance on the affected side with reduced breath sounds and vocal fremitus.
- Progressive hypotension due to reduced venous return and therefore reduced filling of the right ventricle.
- Eventually collapse and cardiac arrest and possibly electromechanical dissociation.

Treatment should be immediate, with insertion of a needle into the pleural space resulting in gas spontaneously escaping from the pleural cavity. A chest drain should then be inserted and connected to an underwater seal.

Acute asthma

This is another medical emergency requiring prompt diagnosis and treatment.

Signs suggestive of a severe asthma attack include:

- Inability of the patient to talk in full sentences due to dyspnoea.
- Patient sitting forward using accessory muscles of respiration—prominent diaphragmatic movements and pursing of the lips on expiration.
- Tachycardia.
- Peak flow 30% of normal or less.
- Pulsus paradoxus—a drop in systolic blood pressure of more than 10 mmHg on inspiration.
- Silent chest due to severe airflow limitation.

Hypercapnoea on blood gas analysis suggests that the patient is becoming exhausted and respiratory arrest may be imminent—this may occur before there is severe hypoxia. The patient should be considered for intubation and artificial ventilation.

Appropriate treatment with intravenous hydrocortisone, oxygen therapy, nebulized bronchodilators and intravenous fluids should be commenced immediately.

Acute left ventricular failure

The detailed management of acute left ventricular failure is discussed in more detail in Chapter 19.

The patient needs urgent treatment or will die from asphyxiation. Classical signs of left ventricular failure can be seen and include:

- Severe dyspnoea.
- Central cyanosis.
- Patient sits upright.
- Bilateral basal fine end-respiratory crepitations (in severe LVF the crepitations extend upwards to fill both lung fields).
- Hypotension secondary to poor left ventricular output (common).

Blood gases show hypoxia and often hypocapnoea due to hyperventilation. There is usually a metabolic acidosis as a result of poor tissue perfusion.

Treatment includes 100% inhaled oxygen via a mask and intravenous frusemide and diamorphine injections.

Pulmonary embolus

This may present in a number of ways, for example:

- Severe dyspnoea.
- Collapse and syncope.
- Hypotension.
- Cardiorespiratory arrest (often with electromechanical dissociation or ventricular fibrillation).

If PE is suspected anticoagulation should be commenced immediately with an intravenous heparin infusion or subcutaneous low molecular weight heparin.

If the patient is cardiovascularly unstable suggesting a massive PE thrombolysis may be administered or emergency pulmonary angiography carried out in an attempt to disrupt the embolus.

Pneumonia

The patient may be pyrexial or even show signs of septic shock (e.g. hypotension, renal failure).

Blood gases may reveal hypoxia, which may be extremely severe in pneumonia caused by *Pneumocystis carinii*.

The chest radiograph may show lobar or patchy consolidation. Radiographic changes may be deceptively mild in mycoplasma or legionella infections.

The most common community-acquired organisms are still streptococci and atypical organisms such as mycoplasma, so appropriate antibiotic therapy should be commenced immediately after blood (and sputum if possible) cultures have been taken.

3. Syncope

Syncope is a loss of conciousness usually due to a reduction in perfusion of the brain.

DIFFERENTIAL DIAGNOSIS OF SYNCOPE

Many conditions may give rise to loss of conciousness—these can be divided into cardiac, vasovagal, circulatory, cerebrovascular, neurological, and metabolic (Fig. 3.1).

HISTORY TO FOCUS ON THE DIFFERENTIAL DIAGNOSIS OF SYNCOPE

The first differentiation to be made is between cardiac and non-cardiac (usually neurological) syncope.

Differentiation depends upon a detailed history of the syncopal episode with particular emphasis on the features outlined below:

The events preceding the syncope should be elucidated:

- Exertion—may precipitate syncope in hypertrophic obstructive cardiomyopathy (HOCM) or aortic stenosis.
- Pain or anxiety—in vasovagal syncope.
- Standing—may precipitate postural hypotension.
- Neck movements—aggravate vertebrobasilar attacks.

Speed of onset of syncope may be:

- Immediate with no warning—classical presentation of Stokes–Adams attacks.
- Rapid with warning—either preceded by lightheadedness (vasovagal) or by an aura (epilepsy).
- Gradual with warning—hypoglycaemia preceded by lightheadedness, nausea, and sweating.

Differential diagnosis of syncope	
System involved	**Pathology**
cardiac	tachyarrhythmia—supraventricular or ventricular bradyarrhythmia—sinus bradycardia, complete or 2nd degree heart block, sinus arrest Stokes–Adams attack—syncope due to transient asystole left ventricular outflow tract obstruction—aortic stenosis, HOCM right ventricular outflow tract obstruction—pulmonary stenosis pulmonary hypertension
vasovagal (simple faint)	after carotid sinus massage and also precipitated by pain, micturition, anxiety; these result in hyperstimulation by the vagus nerve leading to AV node block (and therefore bradycardia, hypotension, and syncope)
vascular	postural hypotension—usually due to antihypertensive drugs or diuretics; also caused by autonomic neuropathy as in diabetes mellitus pulmonary embolus—may or may not be preceded by chest pain septic shock—severe peripheral vasodilatation results in hypotension
cerebrovascular	transient ischaemic attack vertebrobasilar attack
neurological	epilepsy
metabolic	hypoglycaemia

Fig. 3.1 Differential diagnosis of syncope. (See also Fig. 9.3.) (AV, atrioventricular; HOCM, hypertrophic obstructive cardiomyopathy.)

A witness account of the syncope itself, which is very important—indeed no history is complete without one:

- Patient lies still breathing regularly—Stokes–Adams attack (a prolonged Stokes–Adams attack may cause epileptiform movements secondary to cerebral anoxia).
- Patient shakes limbs or has facial twitching and possibly associated with urinary incontinence and tongue biting—epilepsy.
- Patient becomes very pale and grey immediately before collapsing—vasovagal (patients who have cardiac syncope become very pale after collapse before regaining consciousness).

The recovery of conciousness can also be characteristic. If the patient:

- Feels very well soon after episode—a cardiac cause likely.
- Feels washed out and nauseated and takes a few minutes to return to normal—the cause is probably vasovagal.
- Has a neurological deficit—transient cerebral ischaemia (transient ischaemic attack, TIA) or epilepsy is likely.
- Is very drowsy and falls asleep soon after regaining conciousness—epilepsy is probable.

Past medical history

As always a thorough history is needed:

- Any cardiac history is important—ischaemia may precipitate arrhythmias.
- A history of stroke or TIA may suggest a cerebrovascular cause.
- Diabetes mellitus may cause autonomic neuropathy and postural hypotension whereas good control of diabetes mellitus puts the patient at risk of hypoglycaemia.
- A history of head injury may suggest epilepsy secondary to cortical scarring.

Drug history

Important points include the following:

- Antihypertensives and diuretic agents predispose to postural hypotension.
- Class I and class III antiarrhythmics may cause long QT syndrome and predispose to torsades de points—all antiarrhythmic agents may cause bradycardia leading to syncope.
- Some other drugs may also predispose to long QT syndrome.

- Vasodilators precipitate syncope in pulmonary hypertension.

Family history

A family history of sudden death or recurrent syncope may occur in patients who have hypertrophic obstructive cardiomyopathy and also in those rare cases of familial long QT syndrome (Romano–Ward and Jervell–Lange–Nielson syndromes).

A few patients who have epilepsy have a family history.

Social history

Note that:

- Alcohol excess is a risk factor for withdrawal fits.
- Smoking is a risk factor for ischaemic heart disease.

Notes on syncope:
- **Cardiovascular syncope is always accompanied by hypotension.**
- **Syncope with normal blood pressure is likely to have a neurological, cerebrovascular or metabolic cause.**
- **Stokes–Adams attacks are episodes of syncope due to cardiac rhythm disturbance.**
- **Fitting while unconscious is not always caused by epilepsy—it can occur in any patient who has cerebral hypoperfusion or a metabolic disorder (e.g. cardiac syncope or syncope secondary to a pulmonary embolus, cerebrovascular event, hypoglycaemia or alcohol withdrawal).**

EXAMINATION OF PATIENTS WHO PRESENT WITH SYNCOPE

The points to note on examination of the patient who has syncope are summarized in Fig. 3.2, and discussed in turn below.

On inspection:
- Look for any neurological deficit suggestive of a cerebrovascular cause.
- Look for any signs of shock—such as pallor or sweating.

Cardiovascular system

On examination note the following:
- Pulse—any tachy- or bradyarrhythmia and character of pulse (slow rising in aortic stenosis, jerky in HOCM).
- Blood pressure lying and standing to detect postural hypotension (> 20 mmHg drop in blood pressure from lying to standing).
- Jugular venous pulse—cannon waves in complete heart block (due to the atrium contracting against a closed tricuspid valve); prominent a wave in pulmonary hypertension.
- Apex beat—double impulse (HOCM), heaving (aortic stenosis).
- Any murmurs.
- Carotid bruits—indicating carotid artery stenosis and cerebrovascular disease.

- Response to carotid sinus massage—apply unilateral firm pressure over the carotid sinus with the patient in bed and attached to a cardiac monitor. Full resuscitative equipment should be easily accessible. Patients who have carotid sinus hypersensitivity will become very bradycardic and may even become asystolic

Neurological system

This system should be fully examined to detect any residual deficit.

Fingerprick test for blood glucose

This is an easy test and if positive may provide valuable diagnostic information.

INVESTIGATION OF PATIENTS WHO PRESENT WITH SYNCOPE

First-line tests to exclude emergencies are shown in Fig. 3.3.

Blood tests

The following tests should be performed:
- Full blood count—anaemia may be secondary to haemorrhage, which will cause postural hypotension; leucocytosis in sepsis and in the postictal period.

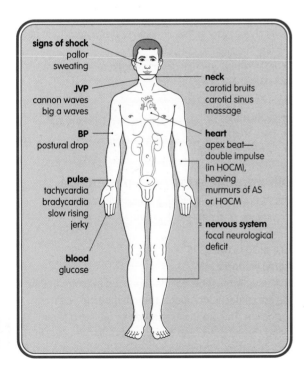

Fig. 3.2 Points to note on examination of a patient presenting with syncope. (AS, aortic stenosis; BP, blood pressure; HOCM, hypertrophic obstructive cardiomyopathy; JVP, jugular venous pressure.)

First-line tests to exclude an emergency syncope	
Test	**Diagnosis**
ECG	look for rhythm distrubance or signs of pulmonary embolus
ECG monitoring on CCU	if suspected cardiac arrhythmia
temperature, Hb, WBC	to look for septic or haemorrhagic cause
blood sugar	to look for hypoglycaemia
CT scan	for possible cerebral infarct or TIA, or intracranial bleed causing fits in a patient who has a recent head injury

Fig. 3.3 First-line tests to exclude an emergency syncope. (CCU, coronary care unit; CT, computed tomography; CXR, chest radiography; ECG, electrocardiography; Hb, haemoglobin; TIA, transient ischaemic attack; WBC, white blood cell count.)

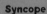
- Electrolytes and renal function—hypokalaemia predisposes towards arrhythmias.
- Calcium—hypocalcaemia is a cause of long QT syndrome.
- Cardiac enzymes—a myocardial infarction may cause sudden arrhythmia.
- Blood glucose.

Electrocardiography

This may show:
- A brady- or tachyarrhythmia.
- Heart block.
- A long QT interval.
- Ischaemia.
- Evidence of a pulmonary embolus.

Holter monitor

This is used to provide a 24- or 48-hour ECG trace to detect arrhythmias and bradycardias (e.g. sick sinus syndrome, intermittent heart block).

Tilt test

This may aid diagnosis:
- Simple tilt produces hypotension and possibly syncope in autonomic denervation.
- Prolonged tilt may provoke vasovagal syncope with bradycardia and hypotension.

Chest radiography

On the chest radiograph:
- There may be cardiomegaly.
- The lung fields may be oligaemic due to a pulmonary embolus.

Echocardiography

This may reveal:
- Aortic stenosis.
- Hypertrophic cardiomyopathy.
- Left atrial enlargement in supraventricular tachycardia.
- Left atrial thrombus in TIA (transthoracic echocardiography cannot reliably diagnose intracardiac thrombus and if this is suspected as a cause of TIA transoesophageal echocardiography is needed).
- Left ventricular abnormalities in ventricular tachycardia or ventricular fibrillation.
- Right ventricular abnormalities in pulmonary hypertension.

Carotid duplex ultrasound scan

To detect carotid atheroma as source of emboli in TIA. This should be performed regardless of whether carotid bruits are present in a patient who is strongly suspected of having TIAs.

Computed tomography scan of the brain

This may reveal areas of previous infarction in a patient who has had a TIA.

Electrophysiological study of the heart

Consider this if cardiac arrhythmia strongly suspected, but not revealed by Holter monitor.

Electroencephalography

This will assist in the diagnosis of epilepsy in selected patients.

SYNCOPE OF RECENT ONSET IN AN ILL PATIENT

The importance of this subject is that this situation represents a medical emergency requiring rapid diagnosis and treatment.

It is necessary in this situation to distinguish between the life-threatening causes:
- Intermittent ventricular tachycardia or fibrillation.
- Intermittent asystole.
- Pulmonary embolus.
- Incipient shock.
- TIA heralding major stroke.
- Hypoglycaemia.

Differentiating features of syncope

The method is to differentiate between cardiac, circulatory, and neurological causes.

Cardiac causes

Aortic stenosis

This usually presents as effort-induced syncope because the left ventricular output is restricted by the outflow restriction. The diagnosis is made by feeling a slow rising carotid pulse and a heaving cardiac impulse in the praecordium. An aortic ejection systolic murmur is present.

Electrocardiography may show left ventricular hypertrophy. Echocardiography reveals the stenotic valve and assessment by Doppler velocity change through the valve (convective acceleration) may give an indication of the severity.

Cardiomyopathies

Hypertrophic obstructive cardiomyopathy can give rise to syncope by obstructing left ventricular outflow on exercise or by giving rise to ventricular tachycardia or fibrillation. This arrhythmic 'sudden death syndrome' can also occur in patients who have non-hypertrophic myocardial dysplasias, and patients who have heart failure (dilated cardiomyopathy).

A wide variety of ECG abnormalities is possible on a resting ECG. Holter monitoring may reveal an intermittent ventricular arrhythmia. Echocardiography reveals hypertrophy, subaortic obstruction, and heart failure (ventricular dilatation). A cardiac electrophysiological study may be necessary in difficult or complex cases.

Long QT syndrome

This may be congenital or drug induced, usually by psychiatric or class III antiarrhythmic drugs (see Chapter 15). The syncope is caused by a self-limiting ventricular tachycardia characterized by a systematically rotating QRS vector (torsade de pointes). The tachycardia and syncope are relieved by rapid pacing or pharmacological sinus tachycardia (e.g. using isoprenaline). The resting non-arrhythmic ECG shows QT prolongation.

Tachyarrhythmias

Syncope is uncommonly due to a supraventricular tachyarrhythmia unless the heart rate is extremely fast. Ventricular tachycardia is more likely to cause syncope because it is accompanied by asynchronous ventricular contraction. If these arrhythmias are not prominent on Holter monitoring, they may be induced during electrophysiological testing.

Bradyarrhythmias

Syncope may occur secondary to a bradyarrhythmia if the cardiac output falls markedly as a consequence of the drop in rate. An ongoing bradyarrhythmia is easily detected using on an ECG (e.g. sinus bradycardia and second degree complete heart block). Some conditions, however, occur intermittently and the ECG may be normal after the syncopal episode, for example:

- Sinus node pauses seen in sick sinus syndrome may cause profound hypotension for a few seconds during the pause, but then revert to sinus rhythm.
- Heart block may occur intermittently with normal sinus rhythm between episodes.

Ambulatory ECG monitoring is therefore needed to capture these episodes. This may be difficult if they are separated by long periods of time.

Circulatory causes

Hypovolaemia

This can present as postural hypotension (i.e. loss of consciousness on standing, relieved by lying flat). This occurs because the blood volume is inadequate, even with an intact baroreflex, to maintain arterial blood pressure in the face of gravity-dependent blood pooling. If this is due to acute haemorrhage there are usually obvious other manifestations such as trauma or haematemesis and melaena. However, internal bleeding can sometimes be difficult to detect. With acute blood loss, the haemoglobin may be normal because there may not have been time for haemodilution to occur.

Septic shock

This causes similar effects by excessive vasodilatation, which prevents baroreflex compensation for postural-dependent blood pooling. However, the patient is usually obviously pyrexial and septic.

Classical postural hypotension

This is due to inadequate baroreflex control. As well as a drop in blood pressure on standing, there may be very little compensatory tachycardia (part of the baroreflex efferent mechanism is to increase heart rate). This can be formally tested by a simple tilt test, during which there is an excessive blood pressure drop and an inadequate tachycardic response.

Obstruction of pulmonary arteries

Obstruction of pulmonary arteries by embolus enters into the differential diagnosis of all cardiovascular emergencies in which syncope is a feature. Chronic thromboembolism or primary pulmonary hypertension can also lead to postural hypotension because the resistance to right ventricular ejection is too high to allow adequate cardiac output when the filling pressure drops on standing.

Cerebrovascular

For full explanation of these syndromes, consult the *Crash Course: Neurology* by A. Bahra and K. Cikurel.

Transient cerebral ischaemia

This often presents to cardiologists because of the known cardiac or arterial causation. These patients show a neurological deficit following their syncope, which recovers with time. There may be repeated episodes. The neurological deficit can often be seen on computed tomography or magnetic resonance scans of the brain. When carotid disease is the source of a cerebral embolus, a bruit may be heard over one or other carotid artery. Even if this is absent, the carotid arteries should be scanned using duplex Doppler to delineate any atheromatous filling defects.

A cardiac source of embolus should be suspected if the patient is in atrial fibrillation.

Left atrial or ventricular thrombus may be difficult to detect by transthoracic echocardiography, in which case a transoesophageal echocardiogram should be performed.

Sometimes TIA is due to an embolus from an infective vegetation of the mitral or aortic valve, or very rarely a left atrial myxoma. These conditions are also investigated by transthoracic and transoesophageal echocardiography.

Patients who have an atrial septal defect may have TIAs secondary to paradoxical emboli (i.e. emboli arising from the right side of the circulation that pass across to the left).

Vertebrobasilar syndrome

This is caused by obstruction of the arteries to the posterior part of the brain (brain stem and cerebellum). The syncope may be preceded by vertigo or dizziness. Precipitation by neck movement is a classical feature in this syndrome when it is associated with cervical spondylosis because the vertebral arteries course within the cervical vertebrae and can get kinked if there is osteoarthritis.

Other neurological causes

Neurological causes without any cardiac or arterial aetiology should be studied in *Crash Course: Neurology*, but epilepsy should always be borne in mind during history taking.

Metabolic causes

For rare causes see *Crash Course: Metabolism and Nutrition* by S. Benyon.

In the common situation of insulin-dependent diabetes mellitus, most patients are inadequately controlled, which leads to more rapid development of heart disease and autonomic neuropathy. Fear of this has driven a few patients to control their diabetes mellitus very obsessively and tightly. These patients tend to experience episodes of loss of consciousness due to hypoglycaemia.

However, hypoglycaemia can occur in any treated diabetic patient and may be precipitated by exercise or reduction in food intake.

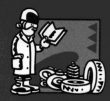

4. Palpitations

Palpitations are an unpleasant awareness of the heart beat. They may be rapid, slow, or just very forceful beats at a normal rate.

Palpitations may be caused by any disorder causing a change in cardiac rhythm or rate and any disorder causing increased stroke volume.

Rapid palpitations

These may be regular or irregular. Regular palpitations may be a sign of:

- Sinus tachycardia.
- Atrial flutter.
- Atrial tachycardia.
- Supraventricular re-entry tachycardia.

Irregularly irregular palpitations may indicate:

- Atrial fibrillation.
- Multiple atrial or ventricular ectopic beats.

Slow palpitations

Patients often describe these as missed beats or forceful beats (after a pause the next beat is often more forceful due to a long filling time and therefore a higher stroke volume). The following may be causes of slow palpitations:

- Sick sinus syndrome.
- Atrioventricular block.
- Occasional ectopics with compensatory pauses.

Disorders causing increased stroke volume

Increased stroke volume may result from:

- Valvular lesions (e.g. mitral or aortic regurgitation).
- High-output states (e.g. pregnancy, thyrotoxicosis or anaemia).

HISTORY TO FOCUS ON THE DIFFERENTIAL DIAGNOSIS OF PALPITATIONS

When taking a history from a patient complaining of palpitations, aim to find answers to the following three questions:

- What is the nature of the palpitations?
- How severe or life-threatening are they?
- What is the likely underlying cause?

Nature of the palpitations

Ask the patient to describe the palpitation by tapping them out (fast, slow, regular, or irregular).

Are the palpitations continuous or intermittent (paroxysmal is the term used for intermittent tachycardias)?

Severity of the palpitations

Determine the severity of the palpitations (i.e. are they associated with complications such as cardiac failure, exacerbation of ischaemic heart disease or thromboembolic events?).

Are the palpitations associated with:

- Syncope, dizziness or shortness of breath?— suggesting that cardiac output is compromised.
- Angina?—suggesting they are causing or being caused by underlying ischaemic heart disease.
- A history of stroke or transient ischaemic attack or limb ischaemia?—suggesting thromboembolic complications of arrhythmia.

Likely underlying causes of palpitation

Are there any features in the history suggestive of the recognized causes of arrhythmias shown in Fig. 4.1.

Fig. 4.1 Features in the history that may suggest the cause of an arrhythmia.

Features in the history suggesting the cause of an arrhythmia	
Features in the history	Cause of arrhythmia
chest pain, breathlessness on exertion, history of myocardial infarction, history of bypass surgery	ischaemic heart disease
tremor, excessive sweating, unexplained weight loss, lethargy, obesity, history of thyroid surgery	thyroid disease
history of rheumatic fever	heart valve disease
peptic ulcer disease, menorrhagia, recent operation	anaemia
alcohol, caffeine, amphetamine, antiarrhythmic agents	proarrhythmic drugs
anxiety	anxiety

EXAMINATION OF PATIENTS WHO HAVE PALPITATIONS

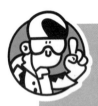

Remember when examining any patient who has a supposedly cardiac problem you must perform a thorough examination of all systems. Cardiac disease can both cause and be caused by disease in other systems so don't get caught out.

Fig. 4.2 summarizes the important points in the examination of a patient who has palpitations, which are outlined below.

General observation

Look for:

- Cyanosis—suggestive of cardiac failure or lung disease (remember that pulmonary embolus is a well-recognized cause of tachyarrhythmia).
- Dyspnoea—suggestive of cardiac failure or lung disease.
- Pallor—suggestive of anaemia.
- Thyrotoxic or myxoedematous facies.

Cardiovascular system
Pulse

Note the rate, rhythm, and character of the pulse at the radial artery (time it for at least 15 s).

Information on the character of the pulse is often more clearly elicited from the carotid pulse, especially features such as:

- A slow rising pulse—due to aortic stenosis.
- A collapsing pulse—due to aortic regurgitation.

A high-volume pulse (due to high-output states and aortic or mitral regurgitation) is often most easily felt at the radial pulse where it is felt as an abnormally strong pulsation.

Blood pressure

This may be low if the patient has palpitations. Hypertension is a cause of atrial fibrillation. A wide pulse pressure is a sign of aortic regurgitation.

Jugular venous pressure

The jugular venous pressure may be elevated if the patient has congestive cardiac failure as a consequence of an uncontrolled tachycardia or who has atrial flutter or fibrillation secondary to pulmonary embolism.

Apex beat

This may be displaced in a patient who has left ventricular failure.

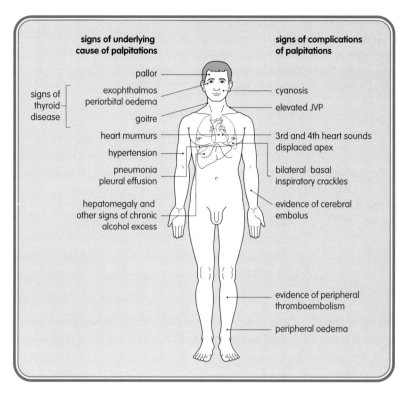

signs of underlying
cause of palpitations

signs of complications
of palpitations

pallor

signs of
thyroid
disease
exophthalmos
periorbital oedema

goitre

heart murmurs

hypertension

pneumonia
pleural effusion

hepatomegaly and
other signs of chronic
alcohol excess

cyanosis

elevated JVP

3rd and 4th heart sounds
displaced apex

bilateral basal
inspiratory crackles

evidence of cerebral
embolus

evidence of peripheral
thromboembolism

peripheral oedema

Fig. 4.2 Important points to note when examining a patient who has palpitations. (CVA, cerebrovascular accident; JVP, jugular venous pressure.)

Heart sounds

A third or fourth heart sound may be heard. Murmurs of mitral or aortic regurgitation are possible causes of high-output state. The murmur of mitral stenosis may be heard in patients who have atrial fibrillation.

Respiratory system

Bilateral basal inspiratory crepitations are heard in a patient who has left ventricular failure. There may be signs of an underlying chest infection (consolidation or effusion), a common cause of palpitations.

Gastrointestinal system

Hepatomegaly and ascites may be signs of congestive cardiac failure or may be signs of alcoholic liver disease—alcohol is one of the most common causes of tachyarrhythmias. Look for other signs of liver disease if this is suspected.

Limbs

On examining the limbs note the following points:
- Peripheral oedema may be a sign of congestive cardiac failure.
- Tremor may be a sign of thyrotoxicosis or alcohol withdrawal.

- Brisk reflexes seen in thyrotoxicosis.
- Weakness—may be a sign of previous cerebral embolus.

INVESTIGATION OF PATIENTS WHO HAVE PALPITATIONS

Blood tests

The following blood tests may aid diagnosis:
- Electrolytes—hypokalaemia is an aggravating factor for most tachyarrhythmias.
- Full blood count—anaemia or a leucocytosis suggesting sepsis may be evident.
- Thyroid function tests.
- Liver function—deranged in congestive cardiac failure or alcoholic liver disease.

Electrocardiography

12-lead electrocardiography

This may enable the diagnosis to be made instantly. However, if the palpitations are intermittent or paroxysmal the ECG may be normal.

There may be signs of the cause of the palpitations on the ECG, for example ischaemia, hypertension, or presence of a delta wave or short PR interval as seen in some congenital causes of paroxysmal tachyarrhythmias such as Wolff–Parkinson–White syndrome (pre-excitation, see p. 116).

24-hour electrocardiography

Monitoring of the ECG for 24 hours may reveal paroxysmal arrhythmias. Patients note down the times that palpitations occur and these can be compared with the recorded ECG at that time. Monitors are available that record the ECG for longer periods of time to diagnose more infrequent episodes.

Exercise electrocardiography

This test may be used to reveal exercise-induced arrhythmias.

Examples of ECGs illustrating atrial fibrillation, atrial flutter, and supraventricular re-entry tachycardia are shown in Fig. 4.3.

Vagotonic manoeuvres

Such manoeuvres include:
- Valsalva manoeuvre.
- Carotid sinus massage.
- Diving reflex.
- Painful stimuli.

These manoeuvres all act by increasing vagal tone, which in turn increases the refractory period of the atrioventricular (AV) node and increases AV node conduction time. By doing this it is possible to differentiate between three common tachyarrhythmias that are sometimes indistinguishable on ECG recording:
- Atrial flutter.
- Atrial fibrillation.
- Supraventricular re-entry tachycardia.

The characteristic features of these tachyarrhythmias are listed in Fig. 4.4.

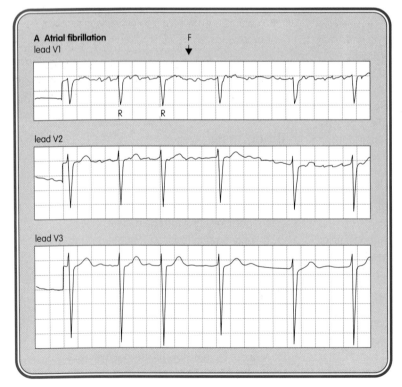

Fig. 4.3A-C Electrocardiograms illustrating atrial fibrillation, atrial flutter, and supraventricular re-entry tachycardia. **(A)** Note the narrow QRS complexes. Fibrillation waves (F) can sometimes be seen. Note the irregularly irregular rhythm and the absence of P waves preceding the QRS complexes. The baseline may show an irregular fibrillating pattern.

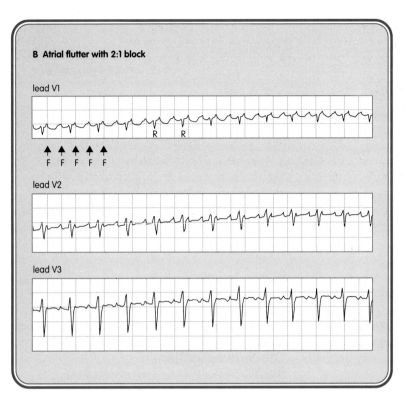

B Atrial flutter with 2:1 block

lead V1

lead V2

lead V3

Fig. 4.3(B) Note the regular rhythm with a rate divisible into 300 (150 beats/min in this case). The P waves are seen in all three leads, but best in V1 at a rate of 300/min. Occasionally the F (flutter) waves form a sawtooth-like pattern (not shown here). Note the F waves at 200 ms intervals (300/min), narrow QRS, and regular RR intervals at 400 ms (150/min).

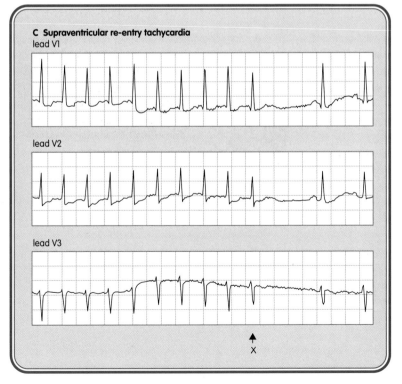

C Supraventricular re-entry tachycardia

lead V1

lead V2

lead V3

Fig. 4.3(C) The rhythm is regular and fast (usually 140–240 beats/min). P waves may be seen and can occur before or after the QRS. Point X shows reversion back to sinus rhythm—note that the following beat has a normal P wave preceding it.

29

Features of atrial fibrillation, atrial flutter, and supraventricular re-entry tachycardia			
Type of tachycardia	Atrial fibrillation	Atrial flutter	Supraventricular re-entry tachycardia
Rate	any rate; pulse deficit if fast	atrial flutter rate is 300/min; the ventricular response is therefore divisible into this (usually 100 or 150/min)	140–260 beats/min
Rhythm	irregularly irregular	regular	regular
Response to adenosine or Valsalva manoeuvre	slowing of ventricular rate reveals underlying lack of P waves	slowing of ventricular rate reveals underlying flutter waves	blocking the AV node may 'break' the re-entry circuit and terminate the tachycardia

Fig. 4.4 Characteristic features of atrial fibrillation, atrial flutter, and supraventricular re-entry tachycardia. (AV node, atrioventricular node.)

Adenosine administration

Adenosine is a purine nucleoside that acts to block the AV node. When administered intravenously it will achieve complete AV block. Its half-life is very short, only a few seconds so this effect is very short-lived.

Side effects of adenosine include bronchospasm, so avoid in asthmatics.

Chest radiography

Look for:
- Evidence of valve disease (e.g. large left atrium and pulmonary vascular congestion in mitral stenosis).
- Evidence of cardiac failure—enlarged heart shadow, pulmonary oedema.
- Kerley B lines.
- Evidence of pulmonary disease—effusion, collapse, or consolidation.

Echocardiography

This will reveal any valvular pathology. It also enables evaluation of left ventricular function.

Electrophysiological study

This is useful in investigating patients suspected of having tachyarrhythmias due to abnormal re-entry pathways. The technique enables localization of the re-entry circuit, which may then be ablated using a radiofrequency thermal electrode placed inside the heart.

Other investigations

A variety of other investigations may be required to identify a suspected cause of the palpitations. These obviously depend upon the clinical evidence, for example:
- Ventilation/perfusion scan if a pulmonary embolus is likely.
- Coronary angiogram if coronary artery disease is suspected.

Whenever investigating, examining or taking a history from a patient with palpitations it is always useful to identify the nature, the severity, and the likely underlying cause of the palpitations. This will enable you to structure your approach and to present your findings in a logical manner.

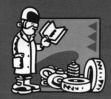

5. Ankle Swelling

Peripheral oedema is caused by an increase in extracellular fluid. The fluid will follow gravity and therefore the ankles are the first part affected in the upright patient.

Ankle swelling is indicative of oedema if there is not a local acute or chronic traumatic cause.

Oedema may be a feature of generalized fluid retention or obstruction of fluid drainage from the lower limbs.

DIFFERENTIAL DIAGNOSIS OF OEDEMA

There are a number of causes of oedema they can be divided into five main groups (Fig. 5.1):

- Cardiac failure—this is due to increased sodium retention secondary to activation of the renin–angiotensin system.
- Hypoalbuminaemia—loss of oncotic pressure within the capillaries causes loss of fluid from the intravascular space.
- Renal impairment—reduction in sodium excretion results in water retention.
- Hepatic cirrhosis—there are a number of mechanisms involved—hypoalbuminaemia (occurs as the hepatic synthetic activity is reduced), peripheral vasodilatation, and activation of the renin–angiotensin system with resulting sodium retention.
- Drugs (e.g. corticosteroids).

Fig. 5.1 Differential diagnosis of ankle oedema.

Differential diagnosis of ankle oedema	
Pathology	Cause
congestive cardiac failure	myocardial infarction, recurrent tachyarrhythmias, (particularly artial fibrillation), hypertensive heart disease, myocarditis, cardiomyopathy due to drugs and toxins, mitral, aortic, or pulmonary valve disease
right heart failure secondary to pulmonary hypertension (cor pulmonale)	chronic lung disease, primary pulmonary hypertension
hypoalbuminaemia	excessive protein loss (due to nephrotic syndrome, extensive burns, protein-losing enteropathy), reduced protein production (due to liver failure), or inadequate protein intake (due to protein–energy malnutrition)
renal disease	any cause of renal impairment (e.g. hypertension, diabetes mellitus, autoimmune disease, infection)
liver cirrhosis	alcohol, hepatitis A, B, C, etc., autoimmune chronic active hepatitis, biliary cirrhosis, Wilson's disease, haemachromatosis, drugs
idiopathic	premenstrual oedema
arteriolar dilatation (exposing the capillaries to high pressure, so increasing intravascular hydrostatic pressure)	dihydropyridine calcium channel blockers (e.g. nifedipine, amlodipine)
sodium retention	Cushing's disease resulting in excessive mineralocorticoid activity, corticosteroids

HISTORY TO FOCUS ON THE DIFFERENTIAL DIAGNOSIS OF ANKLE SWELLING

The first differentiation to be made is between cardiac and non-cardiac oedema. The cause of the oedema is usually revealed by a detailed systems review because there are often symptoms related to the underlying disorder.

Associated breathlessness suggests:

- Pulmonary oedema—this can occur due to cardiac failure or renal failure.
- Chronic lung disease (e.g. chronic obstructive airways disease causes breathlessness).
- Primary and thromboembolic pulmonary hypertension—cause breathlessness and right heart failure.

Other important signs and symptoms include:

- Chest pain and palpitations—suggest underlying cardiac disease (ischaemia or arrhythmias, respectively).
- A history of alcohol or drug abuse or of previous liver disease—suggests a hepatic cause for the oedema.
- Diarrhoea—may be due to a protein-losing enteropathy.

Past medical history

A detailed history of all previous illnesses and operations will provide clues in a patient who has longstanding cardiac, hepatic, or liver disease

Drug history

Important points include the following:

- Some drugs may be renotoxic (e.g. non-steroidal anti-inflammatory agents, angiotensin-converting enzyme inhibitors).
- Some may be hepatotoxic (e.g. methotrexate).
- Dihydropyridine calcium channel blockers cause ankle oedema in some patients.

Social history

Important findings may include:

- Smoking—a risk factor for ischaemic heart disease.
- Intravenous drug abuse—a risk factor for hepatitis.
- Alcohol use—a risk factor for hepatic cirrhosis.

Causes of localized oedema in either the arms or legs include:
- Local venous thrombosis or compression
- Local cellulitis
- Local trauma
- Lymphoedema secondary to obstruction of lymphatic drainage (e.g. secondary to malignancy)

EXAMINATION OF PATIENTS WHO HAVE OEDEMA

A thorough examination of all systems usually reveals the underlying disease.

Cardiovascular system

Check the pulse and blood pressure:

- The pulse is often fast in the patient who has cardiac failure.
- Blood pressure may be low.
- Patients who have chronic renal disease are often hypertensive.

Check the jugular venous pressure (JVP). This is elevated in all patients who have generalized fluid overload and is therefore not a specific sign (only an elevated JVP in the absence of oedema is specific for right ventricular failure).

On examination of the praecordium:

- The apex may be diffuse and laterally displaced in the patient who has cardiac failure.
- There may be a left parasternal heave suggestive of right ventricular strain.
- There may be added third and fourth heart sounds in cardiac failure.
- Audible murmurs may be present suggesting a valvular cause for cardiac failure.

Remember that left ventricular dilatation causes mitral regurgitation due to stretching of the valve ring. Similarly tricuspid regurgitation is often the result of right ventricular enlargement.

Respiratory system

On inspection, consider the following:

- The patient may be tachypnoeic and cyanosed—this may be secondary to cardiac or respiratory disease.
- The lungs may be hyperinflated (due to emphysema) or poorly expansile.

Expansion is reduced in all causes of lung disease, except perhaps primary pulmonary hypertension.

The lung bases may be stony dull indicating bilateral pleural effusions—these are a sign of generalized fluid retention.

Findings on auscultation of the lungs can include:

- Bilateral basal fine inspiratory crepitations suggesting left ventricular failure.
- Coarse crepitations or wheeze, which may be heard in bronchitis or emphysema.
- Mid inspiratory crepitations, which may be heard in pulmonary fibrosis.

Gastrointestinal system

Points to consider on inspection are as follows:

- Does the patient have signs of chronic liver disease such as jaundice, liver flap, spider naevi, gynaecomastia, loss of sexual hair, and testicular atrophy?
- Does the patient have renal failure and look uraemic?

Palpation of the abdomen may reveal ascites in patients who have liver, cardiac, or renal disease. A caput medusae may be evident.

Dipstick the urine—this is part of every examination of the gastrointestinal system. Proteinuria is a feature of nephrotic syndrome and other causes of renal impairment. Haematuria is seen in some diseases causing renal impairment.

Examination of the oedema

Oedema of generalized fluid retention is pitting in nature. To demonstrate this the area in question should be pressed firmly for at least 15 s—there will be an indent in the oedema after this. Be careful: ankle oedema is often tender. The severity of the ankle oedema can be roughly gauged by the extent to which the oedema can be felt up the leg.

Lymphoedema and chronic venous oedema do not 'pit'.

Fig. 5.2 summarizes the findings in patients who have ankle swelling.

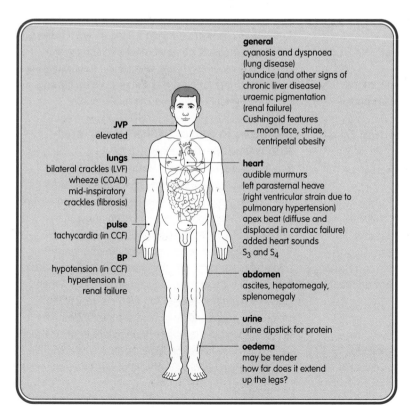

Fig. 5.2 Signs in patients who present with ankle swelling. (BP, blood pressure; CCF, congestive cardiac failure; COAD, chronic obstructive airways disease; JVP, jugular venous pressure; LVF, left ventricular failure.)

general
cyanosis and dyspnoea (lung disease)
jaundice (and other signs of chronic liver disease)
uraemic pigmentation (renal failure)
Cushingoid features — moon face, striae, centripetal obesity

JVP
elevated

lungs
bilateral crackles (LVF)
wheeze (COAD)
mid-inspiratory crackles (fibrosis)

heart
audible murmurs
left parasternal heave (right ventricular strain due to pulmonary hypertension)
apex beat (diffuse and displaced in cardiac failure)
added heart sounds
S_3 and S_4

pulse
tachycardia (in CCF)

BP
hypotension (in CCF)
hypertension in renal failure

abdomen
ascites, hepatomegaly, splenomegaly

urine
urine dipstick for protein

oedema
may be tender
how far does it extend up the legs?

INVESTIGATION OF PATIENTS WHO HAVE OEDEMA

Blood tests

The following blood tests should be considered:

- Full blood count—anaemia is common in chronic renal disease and can precipitate cardiac failure.
- Renal function—this is abnormal in renal disease, but note that patients who have longstanding cardiac or liver disease often have deranged renal function.
- Liver function—this is abnormal in liver disease, but note that hepatic congestion due to cardiac failure also causes abnormal liver function tests.
- Plasma albumin concentration.
- Thyroid function—hyperthyroidism may precipitate cardiac failure.

If Cushing's disease is suspected the following tests are indicated:

- Random serum cortisol.
- Midnight and 9 a.m. serum cortisol—will show loss of diurnal variation.
- Dexamethasone suppression test—short and long.
- 24-hour urine cortisol excretion.

Urine tests

With urine tests, note:

- A 24-hour urine protein excretion test is mandatory if there is no evidence of cardiac disease and the plasma albumin is low.
- Nephrotic syndrome causes loss of at least 3 g protein in 24 hours.

Arterial blood gases

These tests may aid diagnosis:

- Hypoxia may be caused by lung or cardiac disease.
- Carbon dioxide retention is a sign of chronic obstructive airways disease.
- Acidosis can occur with normal oxygen and carbon dioxide (metabolic acidosis) in both liver and renal failure.

Electrocardiography

This may show evidence of tachycardia and old myocardial infarction in a patient who has cardiac failure.

Chest radiography

Chest radiography may help diagnose:

- Cardiomegaly.
- Pulmonary oedema.
- Pleural effusions.
- Lung overexpansion.

Echocardiography

This may show poor ventricular function or valve lesions.

Ultrasound

Regarding ultrasound:

- In a patient who has no evidence of cardiac, renal, or liver disease and bilateral ankle oedema a venous obstruction or external compression must be excluded.
- Doppler ultrasound to detect venous thrombosis and ultrasound of the pelvis to exclude a mass lesion causing compression are appropriate.

IMPORTANT ASPECTS

Salt and water retention

It is important to appreciate that oedema in heart failure is due to generalized salt and water retention, which results from the neurohumoral response to heart failure (see Chapter 19). The symptoms and signs do not therefore differ from those due to generalized salt and water retention in other conditions with similar neurohumoral response. A similar picture is obtained when the salt and water retention is primarily renal in origin.

Increase in extracellular water and intravascular blood volume

Salt and water retention cause an increase in extracellular water and intravascular blood volume. The increase in volume of blood in the heart and central vessels increases pressures, including right atrial pressure. This is appreciated clinically as raised JVP. It can be observed very simply that the appearance of oedema occurs first, and the increase in JVP follows as the central compartment subsequently fills up. When diuretics are administered, the JVP goes down first before the peripheral oedema disappears. Therefore it is incorrect to diagnose right heart failure from a raised JVP in the presence of oedema, but only when the JVP is raised when oedema is absent or has been removed.

Hypertension treated with calcium antagonists

Oedema commonly appears in patients who have hypertension treated with the dihydropyridine calcium antagonists (e.g. nifedipine, amlodipine).

This is due to disturbance of Starling's forces in the tissue, not to general fluid retention. This type of oedema should not be treated with diuretics, which cause electrolyte depletion.

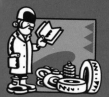

6. Heart Murmur

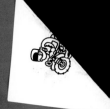

A heart murmur is caused by turbulence of blood flow, which occurs when the velocity of blood is disproportionate to the size of the orifice it is moving through.

DIFFERENTIAL DIAGNOSIS OF A HEART MURMUR

Many conditions can give rise to a murmur:
- Valve lesions—either stenosis or regurgitation of any heart valve.
- Left ventricular outflow obstruction—an example is hypertrophic obstructive cardiomyopathy (HOCM).
- Ventricular septal defect.
- Vascular disorders—coarctation of the aorta, patent ductus arteriosus, arteriovenous malformations (pulmonary or intercostal), venous hum (cervical or hepatic).
- Increased blood flow—normal anatomy, but increased blood flow as in high-output states. Examples of high-output states are anaemia, pregnancy, thyrotoxicosis, or childhood.
- Increased flow across a normal pulmonary valve in atrial and ventricular septal defect.

Cardiac sounds may be confused for murmurs; these include:
- **Third and fourth heart sounds.**
- **Mid-systolic clicks, heard in mitral valve prolapse.**
- **Pericardial friction rub.**

A differential diagnosis of heart murmur is shown in Fig. 6.1.

HISTORY TO FOCUS ON THE DIFFERENTIAL DIAGNOSIS OF A HEART MURMUR

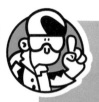

When taking a history from a patient who has a heart murmur, aim to answer the following questions:
- **What is the possible aetiology of the murmur (e.g. infective endocarditis, valve lesion secondary to rheumatic heart disease, high-output state, etc.)?**
- **Are there any complications of valve disease (e.g. cardiac failure, exacerbation of ischaemic heart disease, arrhythmias, syncope, etc.)?**

Presenting complaint

Common presenting complaints include:
- Shortness of breath—suggestive of cardiac failure; also ankle swelling, paroxysmal nocturnal dyspnoea, fatigue.
- Chest pain—due to ischaemic heart disease or atypical chest pain seen in patients who have mitral valve prolapse.
- Syncope—especially seen in patients who have left ventricular outflow obstruction (e.g. aortic stenosis or HOCM).
- Fever, rigors, and malaise—common presenting complaints in patients who have infective endocarditis.
- Palpitations—for example mitral valve disease is associated with atrial fibrillation.

Past medical history

Aim to elicit any history of cardiac disease with particular emphasis on possible causes of a murmur:

- History of rheumatic fever in childhood.
- Previous cardiac surgery.
- Myocardial infarction in past—may cause ventricular dilatation and therefore functional regurgitation or rupture or dysfunction of papillary muscle leading to mitral regurgitation.
- Family history of cardiac problems or sudden death—as may occur for patients who have HOCM.

- Recent dental procedures or operations—may be a cause of infective endocarditis.

Social history

Ask in particular about:

- Smoking—an important risk factor for ischaemic heart disease.
- Alcohol intake—if excessive may result in dilated cardiomyopathy.
- History of intravenous drug abuse.

Differential diagnosis of heart murmur			
Phase of cardiac cycle	Nature of murmur	Valve lesion	Cause of valve lesion
systolic	ejection systolic	aortic stenosis (AS)	valvular stenosis, congenital valvular abnormality, rheumatic fever, supravalvular stenosis, subvalvular stenosis, senile valvular calcification
		aortic sclerosis	aortic valve roughening
		HOCM	left ventricular outflow tract (subaortic) stenosis
		increased flow across normal valve	high output states (e.g. anaemia, fever, pregnancy, thyrotoxicosis)
	pansystolic	mitral regurgitation (MR)	functional MR due to dilatation of mitral valve annulus valvular MR: rheumatic fever, infective endocarditis, mitral valve prolapse, chordal rupture, papillary muscle infarct
		tricuspid regurgitation (TR)	functional TR valvular TR: rheumatic fever, infective endocarditis
		VSD with left to right shunt	congenital, septal infarct (acquired)
diastolic	early diastolic	aortic regurgitation (AR)	functional AR: dilatation of valve ring, aortic dissection, cystic medial necrosis (Marfan syndrome) valvular AR: rheumatic fever, infective endocarditis, bicuspid aortic valve
		pulmonary regurgitation (PR)	functional PR: dilatation of valve ring, Marfan syndrome, pulmonary hypertension valvular PR: rheumatic fever, carcinoid, Fallot's tetralogy
	mid-diastolic	mitral stenosis (MS)	rheumatic fever, congenital
		tricuspid stenosis (TS)	rheumatic fever
		left and right atrial myxomas	tumour obstruction of valve orifice in diastole
continuous		PDA	congenital
		arteriovenous fistula	
		cervical venous hum	

Fig. 6.1 Differential diagnosis of heart murmur. (HOCM, hypertrophic obstructive cardiomyopathy; PDA, patent ductus arteriosus; VSD, ventricular septal defect.)

EXAMINATION OF PATIENTS WHO HAVE A HEART MURMUR

General observation

Look for signs of cardiac failure (i.e. dyspnoea, cyanosis, or oedema). Look also for clues indicating the cause of the murmur:

- Anaemia—may cause a high-output state or be caused by infective endocarditis.
- Scars of previous cardiac surgery—median sternotomy, thoracotomy, or valvuloplasty scars.

Examine the eyes for retinal haemorrhages (Roth's spots) and conjunctival haemorrhages. These are signs of infective endocarditis.

Fig. 6.2 gives a summary of the findings on examination of a patient who has a heart murmur.

Hands

Look for peripheral stigmas of infective endocarditis:

- Splinter haemorrhages—more than five is pathological.

- Osler's nodes (purplish raised papules on finger pulps).
- Janeway lesions (erythematous non-tender lesions on the thenar eminence).
- Finger clubbing.

Cardiovascular system

Pulse

Examine the pulse both at the radial site and the internal carotid artery. Examples of abnormal pulse due to valvular disease include:

- Slow rising or plateau pulse in aortic stenosis.
- Collapsing or waterhammer pulse in aortic regurgitation or patent ductus arteriosus.
- Bisferiens pulse in mixed aortic valve disease.
- A jerky pulse in HOCM.

Blood pressure

This may also give important clues:

- A narrow pulse pressure associated with hypotension is a sign of severe aortic stenosis.
- A wide pulse pressure may be seen in aortic regurgitation or high-output states.

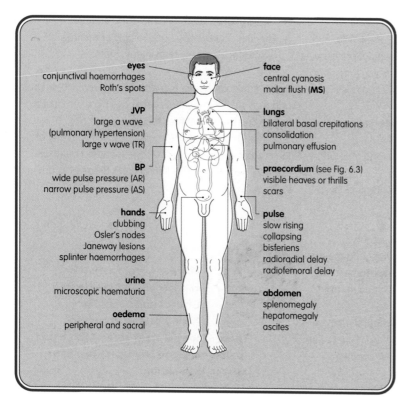

Fig. 6.2 Possible findings in a patient who has a heart murmur. (AS, aortic stenosis; AR, aortic regurgitation; MS, mitral stenosis; TR, tricuspid regurgitation.)

eyes
conjunctival haemorrhages
Roth's spots

JVP
large a wave
(pulmonary hypertension)
large v wave (TR)

BP
wide pulse pressure (AR)
narrow pulse pressure (AS)

hands
clubbing
Osler's nodes
Janeway lesions
splinter haemorrhages

urine
microscopic haematuria

oedema
peripheral and sacral

face
central cyanosis
malar flush (**MS**)

lungs
bilateral basal crepitations
consolidation
pulmonary effusion

praecordium (see Fig. 6.3)
visible heaves or thrills
scars

pulse
slow rising
collapsing
bisferiens
radioradial delay
radiofemoral delay

abdomen
splenomegaly
hepatomegaly
ascites

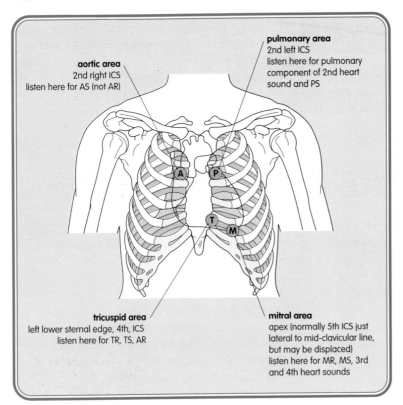

Fig. 6.3 Praecordium, illustrating the position of valve areas. (AR, aortic regurgitation; AS, aortic stenosis; ICS, intercostal space; MR, mitral regurgitation; MS, mitral stenosis; PS, pulmonary stenosis; TR, tricuspid regurgitation; TS, tricuspid stenosis.)

aortic area
2nd right ICS
listen here for AS (not AR)

pulmonary area
2nd left ICS
listen here for pulmonary component of 2nd heart sound and PS

tricuspid area
left lower sternal edge, 4th, ICS
listen here for TR, TS, AR

mitral area
apex (normally 5th ICS just lateral to mid-clavicular line, but may be displaced)
listen here for MR, MS, 3rd and 4th heart sounds

Jugular venous pressure

Remember the patient must be at 45 degrees with the neck muscles relaxed. The jugular venous pressure is measured as the height of the visible pulsation vertically from the sternal angle. Possible findings include:

- An elevated jugular venous pressure in congestive cardiac failure.
- Large a waves in pulmonary stenosis and pulmonary hypertension.
- Large v waves—a sign of tricuspid regurgitation.

Praecordium

Remember to look for scars of previous surgery.

On palpation the apex beat is the lowest and most lateral point at which the cardiac impulse can be felt. Possible abnormalities in a patient who has a murmur include:

- Displaced apex beat—due to mitral regurgitation and aortic regurgitation.
- Double apical impulse—due to HOCM, also left ventricular aneurysm.
- Tapping apex beat—due to mitral stenosis.

- Heaving apex beat—due to aortic stenosis.
- Thrusting apex beat—due to aortic or mitral regurgitation or any high-output state.

Right ventricular heave is a sign of right ventricular strain and may be felt in patients who have right ventricular failure due to mitral valve disease.

Thrills (or palpable murmurs) may be felt in any of the cardiac areas where the corresponding murmurs are best heard). The position of valve areas are shown in Fig. 6.3.

Murmurs from valves on the left side of the heart (mitral and aortic) are heard best in expiration. Those from the right side of the heart (pulmonary and tricuspid) are heard best in inspiration.

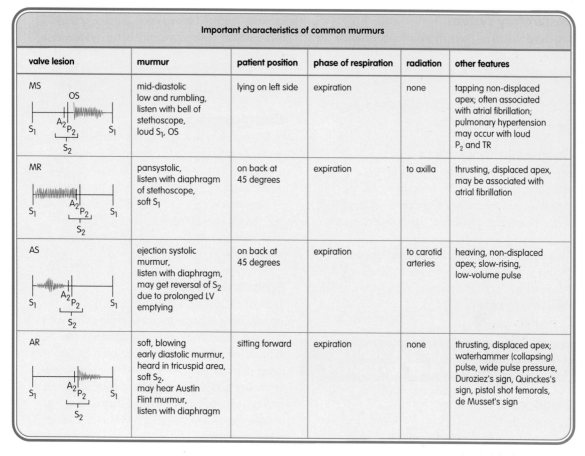

valve lesion	murmur	patient position	phase of respiration	radiation	other features
MS	mid-diastolic low and rumbling, listen with bell of stethoscope, loud S₁, OS	lying on left side	expiration	none	tapping non-displaced apex; often associated with atrial fibrillation; pulmonary hypertension may occur with loud P₂ and TR
MR	pansystolic, listen with diaphragm of stethoscope, soft S₁	on back at 45 degrees	expiration	to axilla	thrusting, displaced apex, may be associated with atrial fibrillation
AS	ejection systolic murmur, listen with diaphragm, may get reversal of S₂ due to prolonged LV emptying	on back at 45 degrees	expiration	to carotid arteries	heaving, non-displaced apex; slow-rising, low-volume pulse
AR	soft, blowing early diastolic murmur, heard in tricuspid area, soft S₂, may hear Austin Flint murmur, listen with diaphragm	sitting forward	expiration	none	thrusting, displaced apex; waterhammer (collapsing) pulse, wide pulse pressure, Duroziez's sign, Quinckes's sign, pistol shot femorals, de Musset's sign

Table title: Important characteristics of common murmurs

Fig. 6.4 Important characteristics of common murmurs. The second heart sound (S₂) has two components —A₂ (aortic valve closure) and P₂ (pulmonary valve closure). (AS, aortic stenosis; AR, aortic regurgitation; MR, mitral regurgitation; MS, mitral stenosis; OS, opening snap; S₁, first heart sound; TR, tricuspid regurgitation.)

It is important to know these important characteristics for each of the common murmurs:

- Location at which to listen for the murmur.
- Position of the patient for each murmur.
- Phase of respiration during which each murmur is best heard.
- Nature of the murmur and where it radiates.

Characteristics of common murmurs are listed in Fig. 6.4.

Peripheral vascular system

All peripheral pulses should be palpated.

Radioradial delay and radiofemoral delay may be found with coarctation of the aorta. Also seen in this condition is discrepancy in the blood pressure taken in each arm. It is important to look for these signs as part of the cardiovascular examination.

Peripheral oedema

This may be elicited by applying firm pressure for at least 15 s.

Respiratory system

The chest should be carefully examined. Possible findings include:

- Bilateral basal fine end-inspiratory crepitations —suggests pulmonary oedema.
- Evidence of respiratory tract infection—sepsis may cause a high-output state.

Gastrointestinal system

Important findings include:

- Hepatomegaly or ascites, seen in right-sided heart failure or congestive cardiac failure.
- Splenomegaly, a feature of infective endocarditis.

Dipstick test of the urine should always be performed as part of the bedside examination. Microscopic haematuria is a common finding in patients who have infective endocarditis.

INVESTIGATION OF PATIENTS WHO HAVE A HEART MURMUR

Blood tests

These include:

- Full blood count—anaemia may be seen as a sign of chronic disease in a patient who has infective endocarditis and is also a cause of hyperdynamic state; a leucocytosis is also a feature of infective endocarditis.
- Urea, creatinine, and electrolytes—may be deranged in patients who have cardiac failure as a result of poor renal perfusion or diuretic therapy.
- Liver function tests—these may be abnormal in patients who have hepatic congestion secondary to cardiac failure.
- Blood cultures—at least three sets should be taken before commencement of antibiotic therapy in all patients in whom infective endocarditis is suspected.
- ESR and C-reactive protein—these are markers of inflammation or infection and are useful in monitoring treatment of infective endocarditis.

Chest radiography

This may reveal an abnormal cardiac shadow (e.g. large left atrium and prominent pulmonary vessels in mitral stenosis, enlarged left ventricle in mitral or aortic regurgitation, or the abnormal aortic shadow in coarctation).

Abnormality in the lung fields may also be seen (e.g. pulmonary oedema, pulmonary effusion).

Electrocardiography

The 12-lead ECG may give useful information:

- Atrial fibrillation may be a sign of mitral valve disease.
- Left ventricular strain pattern may be seen in aortic stenosis.
- P mitrale may be seen in the ECG if there is pulmonary hypertension secondary to valve disease (as occurs in severe mitral stenosis).

Echocardiography

Transthoracic echocardiography

Transthoracic echocardiography enables the valves to be visualized and pressure gradients across them to be assessed. Left ventricular function and pulmonary artery pressure can be estimated. The presence of ventricular septal defect or patent ductus arteriosus may be more accurately assessed by cardiac catheterization, but they may be visualized using echocardiography.

Transoesophageal echocardiography

Transoesophageal echocardiography is very useful because it gives very detailed information on structures that are difficult to see using transthoracic echocardiography. Examples of its uses include:

- Assessment of prosthetic valves.
- Detailed evaluation of the mitral valve before mitral valve repair.

Cardiac catheterization

Before valve replacement this is performed to obtain information about the:

- Presence of coexisting coronary artery disease.
- Degree of pulmonary hypertension in patients who have mitral valve disease.

This investigation can also be used to assess the severity of the left-to-right shunt in patients who have ventricular or atrial septal defects.

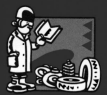

7. High Blood Pressure

A person is hypertensive if three sets of blood pressure measurements taken over at least a 3-month period are higher than 140/90 mmHg. If the blood pressure is found to be very high, however, three such measurements may not be required to make the diagnosis.

DIFFERENTIAL DIAGNOSIS

Systemic hypertension may be classified as:
- Primary (essential) hypertension, for which there is no identified cause. This accounts for 95% of cases.
- Secondary hypertension, for which there is a clear cause (Fig. 7.1).

Causes of secondary hypertension	
Mechanism	**Pathology**
renal	renal parenchymal disease (e.g. chronic atrophic pyelonephritis, chronic glomerulonephritis), renal artery stenosis, renin-producing tumours, primary sodium retention
endocrine	acromegaly, hypo- and hyperthyroidism, hypercalcaemia, adrenal cortex disorders (e.g. Cushing's disease, Conn's syndrome, congenital adrenal hyperplasia), adrenal medulla disorders e.g. phaeochromocytoma
vascular disease	coarctation of the aorta
other	hypertension of pregnancy, carcinoid syndrome
increased intravascular volume	polycythaemia (primary or secondary)
drugs	alcohol, oral contraceptives, monoamine oxidase inhibitors, glucocorticoids
psychogenic	stress

Fig. 7.1 Causes of secondary hypertension.

HISTORY TO FOCUS ON THE DIFFERENTIAL DIAGNOSIS OF HIGH BLOOD PRESSURE

Presenting complaint

Hypertensive patients are often asymptomatic. Occasionally they complain of headaches, tinnitus, recurrent epistaxis, or dizziness. In this situation a detailed systems review may reveal clues as to a possible cause of hypertension:
- Weight loss or gain, tremor, hair loss, heat intolerance, or feeling cold may suggest the presence of thyroid disease.
- Paroxysmal palpitations, sweating, headaches, or collapse may indicate the possibility of a phaeochromocytoma.

Ask the patient about symptoms that may indicate the presence complications of hypertension such as:
- Dyspnoea, orthopnoea, or ankle oedema suggesting cardiac failure.
- Chest pain indicating ischaemic heart disease.
- Unilateral weakness or visual disturbance (either persistent or transient) suggesting cerebrovascular disease.

Past medical history

To gain information about a condition that has so many varied causes it is crucial to ask about all previous illnesses and operations. Examples include:
- Recurrent urinary tract infections, especially in childhood, may lead to chronic pyelonephritis, a common cause of renal failure.
- A history of asthma may reveal chronic corticosteroid intake, leading to Cushing's syndrome.
- Thyroid surgery in the past.
- Evidence of peripheral vascular disease (e.g. leg claudication or previous vascular surgery may suggest the possibility of underlying renovascular disease).

Drug history

A careful history of all drugs being taken regularly is needed including use of proprietary analgesics (e.g. aspirin, nonsteroidal anti-inflammatory drugs; a possible cause of renal disease).

Family history

Essential hypertension is a multifactorial disease requiring both genetic and environmental inputs. A family history of hypertension is therefore not an uncommon finding in these patients. Some secondary causes of hypertension have a genetic component:

- Adult polycystic kidney disease is an autosomal dominant condition associated with hypertension renal failure and cerebral artery aneurysms.
- Phaeochromocytoma may occur as part of a multiple endocrine neoplasia syndrome associated with medullary carcinoma of the thyroid and hyperparathyroidism (MEN 2, autosomal dominant).

Social history

Smoking, like hypertension, is a risk factor for ischaemic heart disease. Excessive alcohol intake may cause hypertension.

EXAMINATION OF PATIENTS WHO HAVE HIGH BLOOD PRESSURE

When performing the examination, look for:

- Signs of end-organ damage (i.e. cardiac failure, ischaemic heart disease, peripheral artery disease, cerebrovascular disease and renal impairment).
- Signs of an underlying cause of hypertension.

Blood pressure

Important points to note are:

- Patient should be seated comfortably—preferably for 5 min before measurement of blood pressure in a quiet warm setting.
- Correct cuff size should be used—if too small a spuriously high reading will result.
- The manometer should be correctly calibrated.
- Bladder should be inflated to 20 mmHg above systolic blood pressure.
- Systolic blood pressure is recorded as the point during bladder deflation where regular sounds can be heard. Systolic blood pressure can also be measured as the pressure at which the palpated distal pulse disappears.
- Diastolic blood pressure is recorded as the point at which the sounds disappear (Korotkoff phase V). In children and pregnant women muffling of the sounds is used as the diastolic blood pressure (Korotkoff phase IV).

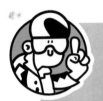

When performing the initial blood pressure measurements measure blood pressure in both arms. A marked difference suggests coarctation of the aorta.

The blood pressure in some patients goes up when they see a doctor—this is 'white coat hypertension'.

Ambulatory blood pressure monitoring is available at some hypertension clinics.

Cardiovascular examination

Examine the pulses, considering the following:

- Rate—tachycardia or bradycardia may indicate underlying thyroid disease.
- Rhythm—atrial fibrillation may occur as a result of hypertensive heart disease.
- Symmetry—compare the pulses, radioradial delay is a sign of coarctation as is the finding of abnormally weak foot pulses.
- Weak or absent peripheral pulses along with cold extremities suggest peripheral vascular disease.

Jugular venous pressure may be elevated in congestive cardiac failure, a complication of hypertension.

A displaced apex is seen in left ventricular failure due to dilatation of the left ventricle.

Mitral regurgitation may occur secondary to dilatation of the valve ring that occurs during left ventricular dilatation.

In patients who have coarctation bruits may be heard over the scapulas and a systolic murmur may be heard below the left clavicle.

Respiratory system

Bilateral basal crepitations of pulmonary oedema may be heard on examination of the respiratory system.

Gastrointestinal system

Hepatomegaly and ascites may be seen in cases with congestive cardiac failure. Abdominal aortic aneurysm must be examined for because it is a manifestation of generalized atherosclerosis. Palpable kidneys may be evident in individuals who have polycystic kidney disease. A renal artery bruit may be heard in cases with renal artery stenosis.

Limbs

Peripheral oedema is a sign of congestive cardiac failure or underlying renal disease.

Eyes

Hypertensive retinopathy

A detailed examination of the fundi is crucial in all patients who have hypertension because it provides valuable information about the severity of the hypertension (Fig. 7.2). Patients exhibiting grade III or IV hypertensive retinopathy have accelerated or malignant hypertension and need urgent treatment.

Fig. 7.3 highlights the features of the different grades of hypertensive retinopathy.

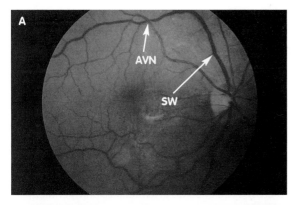

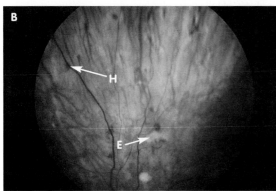

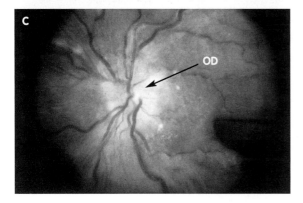

Fig. 7.2 Stages of hypertensive retinopathy. **(A)** Grade II, showing silver wiring (SW) and arteriovenous nipping (AVN) where an artery crossing above a vein causes apparent compression of the underlying vein. **(B)** Grade III, showing evidence of haemorrhages (H) and exudates (E). **(C)** Papilloedema—the optic disc (OD) is swollen and oedematous—a sign of malignant hypertension.

Features of hypertension	
Grade	Features
I	narrowing of the arteriolar lumen occurs giving the classical 'silver wiring' effect
II	sclerosis of the adventitia and thickening of the muscular wall of the arteries leads to compression of underlying veins and 'arteriovenous nipping'
III	rupture of small vessels leading to haemorrhages and exudates
IV	papilloedema (plus signs of grades I–IV)

Fig. 7.3 Features of hypertensive retinopathy on ophthalmoscopy.

Other findings on examination

When examining a patient who has a disorder that has many possible causes, a thorough examination of all systems is vital. Remember to look out for signs of thyroid disease, Cushing's disease, acromegaly, renal impairment, etc.

INVESTIGATION OF PATIENTS WHO HAVE HIGH BLOOD PRESSURE

Look for evidence of end-organ damage and possible underlying causes.

Blood tests

The following blood tests may help in the diagnosis:

- Electrolytes and renal function—many patients who have hypertension may be treated with diuretics and therefore may have hypokalaemia or hyponatraemia as a result. Renal impairment either as a result of hypertension or its treatment must be excluded.
- Full blood count—polycythaemia may be present. Macrocytosis may be seen in hypothyroidism; anaemia may be a result of chronic renal failure.
- Blood glucose—elevated blood glucose may be seen in diabetes mellitus or in Cushing's disease.
- Thyroid function.

- Blood lipid profile—like hypertension, an important risk factor for ischaemic heart disease.

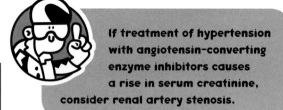

If treatment of hypertension with angiotensin-converting enzyme inhibitors causes a rise in serum creatinine, consider renal artery stenosis.

Urinalysis

Look for protein casts or red blood cells—a sign of underlying renal disease.

Electrocardiography

There may be evidence of left ventricular hypertrophy. Features of left ventricular hypertrophy, shown in Fig. 7.4, are:

- Tall R waves in lead V6 (>25 mm).
- R wave in V5 plus S wave in V2 greater than 50 mm.
- Deep S wave in lead V2.
- Inverted T waves in lateral leads (i.e. I, AVL, V5, and V6).

There may be evidence of an old myocardial infarction or of rhythm disturbance especially atrial fibrillation.

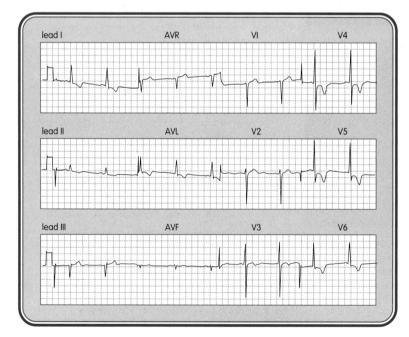

Fig. 7.4 Electrocardiographic features of left ventricular hypertrophy (LVH). Note the three cardinal features indicating LVH —R wave in V5 plus S wave in V2 exceeds 7 large squares; the R wave in V6 and S wave in V2 are greater than 5 large squares; T wave inversion in lateral leads V4–V6.

Chest radiography

Look for:

- An enlarged left ventricle—seen on the chest radiograph as an enlarged cardiac shadow. The normal ratio of cardiac width to thoracic width is 1:2.
- Evidence of coarctation of the aorta—this is seen as poststenotic dilatation of the aorta with an indentation above producing the reversed figure three, along with rib notching due to dilatation of the posterior intercostal arteries.

Echocardiography

This investigation is used to:

- Reveal left ventricular hypertrophy.
- Reveal poor left ventricular function.
- Show any areas of left ventricular hypokinesia suggestive of old myocardial infarction.

Investigations to exclude secondary hypertension

The above investigations may point to possible underlying causes of secondary hypertension, but are not exhaustive. It would not, however, be cost-effective to investigate all hypertensive patients for these disorders because over 95% of cases of hypertension are primary.

Careful selection of patients who are more likely to have secondary hypertension is therefore needed before embarking on more detailed and invasive investigations.

Secondary hypertension is more likely in patients who are under 35 years of age and also in patients who have:

- Symptoms of malignant hypertension (i.e. severe headaches, nausea and vomiting, blood pressure >180/100 mmHg, papilloedema).
- Evidence of end-organ damage (i.e. grade III or IV retinopathy, raised serum creatinine, cardiac failure).
- Signs of secondary causes (e.g. hypokalaemia in the absence of diuretics, signs of coarctation, abdominal bruit, symptoms of phaeochromocytoma, family history of renal disease or stroke at a young age).
- Poorly controlled blood pressure despite medical therapy.

Investigations for secondary hypertension are listed in Fig. 7.5.

Failure of hypertension to respond to treatment may be because there is an underlying secondary cause or because of lack of compliance with therapy

Investigation of secondary hypertension		
Underlying cause	**Investigation**	**Notes/Result**
renal parenchymal disease	24-hour creatinine clearance 24-hour protein excretion renal ultrasound renal biopsy	↓ ↑ bilateral small kidneys in some cases
renal artery stenosis	renal ultrasound radionucleotide studies using DTPA renal angiography or MRI angiography	often asymmetrical kidneys decreased uptake on affected side; this effect is highlighted by administration of an ACE inhibitor
phaeochromocytoma	24-hour urine catecholamines CT scan of abdomen MIBG scan	↑, VMA measurements now rarely used tumour is often large to identify extra-adrenal tumours (seen in 10% cases)
Cushing's disease	24-hour urinary free cortisol dexamethasone suppression test 0900 and 2400 blood cortisol adrenal CT scan pituitary MRI scan chest X-ray	↑ low-dose 48-hour test initially, high-dose test to rule out ectopic source of ACTH reveals loss of circadian rhythm in Cushing's disease may show oat cell carcinoma of bronchus (ectopic ACTH)

Fig. 7.5 Investigation of secondary hypertension. (ACE, angiotensin converting enzyme; ACTH, adrenocorticotrophic hormone; CT, computed tomography; MIBG, meta-iodobenzylguanidine; MRI, magnetic resonance imaging; VMA, vanillylmandelic acid.)

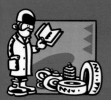

8. Fever Associated with a Cardiac Symptom or Sign

DIFFERENTIAL DIAGNOSIS

Some very serious and potentially fatal cardiac conditions are accompanied by fever. It is therefore important to have at hand a working list of differential diagnoses when presented with such a case.

In the viva a well-presented list of differential diagnoses implies that you can think laterally and adapt your knowledge of cardiac conditions to fit a clinical scenario.

Whenever presenting a list of differential diagnoses start with either the most dangerous or the most common disorder first. Leave the rare conditions to the end (even though these are invariably the ones that immediately spring to mind.)

The differential diagnosis includes:
- Infective endocarditis (bacterial or fungal infection within the heart).
- Myocarditis (involvement of the myocardium in an inflammatory process, which is usually infectious).
- Pericarditis (inflammation of the pericardium, which may be infective, postmyocardial infarction, or autoimmune).
- Other rare conditions, such as cardiac myxoma.

The fever may be of non-cardiac origin.

Rare conditions
Cardiac myxomas:
- Are benign primary tumours of the heart.
- Are most often located in the atria.
- May present with a wide variety of symptoms (e.g. dyspnoea, fever, weight loss).
- Can cause complications such as thromboembolic phenomena or sudden death.
- Are diagnosed by echocardiography.
- Are treated with anticoagulation to prevent thromboembolic phenomena and resection (they may recur if incompletely resected).

HISTORY TO FOCUS ON THE DIFFERENTIAL DIAGNOSIS OF FEVER

When presented with a set of symptoms that cover a potentially huge set of differential diagnoses it is important to be systematic.

Remember that sepsis is a common cause of atrial fibrillation and flutter. Patients who have sepsis may therefore present with fever and palpitations.

Presenting complaint
Common presenting complaints include:
- Fever—ask when it started and whether the patient can think of any precipitating factors (e.g. an operation or dental work).

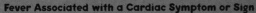

Important features of ischaemic and pericarditic pain.		
Condition	Pericarditis	Ischaemia
Location	praecordium	retrosternal +/− radiation to left arm, throat or jaw
Quality	sharp, pleuritic (may be dull)	pressure pain (usually builds up)
Duration	hours to days	minutes, usually resolving (occasionally lasts hours)
Relationship to exercise	no	yes unless unstable angina or myocardial infarction
Relationship to posture	worse when recumbent, relieved when sitting forward	usually no effect

Fig. 8.1 Important features of ischaemic and pericarditic pain.

- Chest pain—to differentiate between for example, ischaemic and pericarditic pain establish the exact nature of the pain, where it radiates, duration, and exacerbating factors (Fig. 8.1).
- Palpitations—ask about rate and rhythm to obtain information about the likely nature of the palpitations. Also ask about the possible complications of palpitations (e.g. dyspnoea, angina, dizziness).

Past medical history

It is crucial to obtain a detailed past medical history. In particular the following aspects of the past medical history are important in these patients:

- Recent dental work—this is a common source of bacteraemia and cause of infective endocarditis.
- Recent operations—these may also cause transient bacteraemia (e.g. gastrointestinal surgery, genitourinary surgery or even endoscopic investigations).
- History of rheumatic fever—although rare in the developed world now, this condition was common in the early 20th century and is the cause of valve damage in many elderly patients. Such abnormal valves are vulnerable to colonization by bacteria.
- Previous myocardial infarction—a possible cause of pericarditis and Dressler's syndrome (a non-specific, possibly autoimmune inflammatory response to cardiac necrosis in surgery).
- Recent viral infection (e.g. a sore throat or a cold) —myocarditis and pericarditis are commonly caused by viral infection.

Drug history

Ask about any recent antibiotics taken—obtain exact details of drugs and doses.

Remember that some drugs may cause pericarditis, for example penicillin (associated with hypereosinophilia), hydralazine, procainamide, and isoniazid.

Social history

Ask about:

- History of intravenous drug abuse, which is a risk factor for infective endocarditis.
- Risk factors for human immunodeficiency virus infection, which may be associated with infection due to unusual organisms.
- Smoking, a common cause for recurrent chest infection or myocardial infarction.

EXAMINATION OF PATIENTS WHO HAVE A FEVER ASSOCIATED WITH A CARDIAC SYMPTOM OR SIGN

Fig. 8.2 highlights the important features on examination of a patient who has fever and a cardiac sign or symptom.

Temperature

If using a mercury thermometer shake it well before use and leave it in the mouth for 3 full minutes.

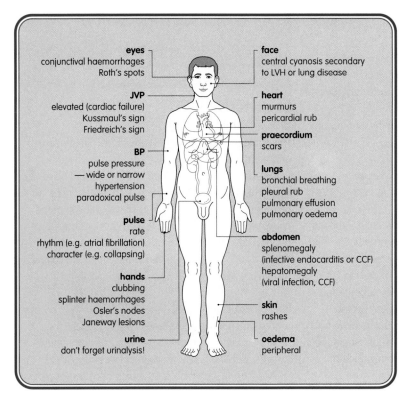

Fig. 8.2 Important signs in a patient who has fever and a cardiac symptom or sign. (CCF, congestive cardiac failure; JVP, jugular venous pressure.)

eyes
conjunctival haemorrhages
Roth's spots

face
central cyanosis secondary to LVH or lung disease

JVP
elevated (cardiac failure)
Kussmaul's sign
Friedreich's sign

heart
murmurs
pericardial rub

praecordium
scars

BP
pulse pressure
— wide or narrow
hypertension
paradoxical pulse

lungs
bronchial breathing
pleural rub
pulmonary effusion
pulmonary oedema

pulse
rate
rhythm (e.g. atrial fibrillation)
character (e.g. collapsing)

abdomen
splenomegaly
(infective endocarditis or CCF)
hepatomegaly
(viral infection, CCF)

hands
clubbing
splinter haemorrhages
Osler's nodes
Janeway lesions

skin
rashes

urine
don't forget urinalysis!

oedema
peripheral

Hands

Look for signs of infective endocarditis:

- Clubbing.
- Osler's nodes (tender purplish nodules on the finger pulps).
- Janeway lesions (erythematous areas on palms).
- Splinter haemorrhages—up to four can be considered to be normal. The most common cause for a lesion that has the same appearance as a splinter haemorrhage is trauma, so they are common in keen gardeners.

All these are signs of vasculitis and may be found in other conditions causing vasculitis (e.g. autoimmune disease).

Facies

Look for:

- Conjunctival haemorrhages and Roth's spots (retinal haemorrhages)—both signs of infective endocarditis.
- Central cyanosis—this may be a sign of a chest infection or cardiac failure.
- A vasculitic rash (e.g. the butterfly rash of systemic lupus erythematosus).

Cardiovascular system
Pulse

Check the:

- Rate and rhythm—may reveal underlying tachyarrhythmia (e.g. atrial fibrillation or, more commonly sinus tachycardia—a common finding in a patient who has pyrexia.
- Quality of pulse—may reveal an underlying valve abnormality (e.g. waterhammer or collapsing pulse suggesting aortic regurgitation caused by endocarditis affecting the aortic valve).

Blood pressure

Hypotension may be found suggesting septic shock or cardiac failure.

A large pericardial effusion causing tamponade may result in pulsus paradoxus, which is an exaggeration of the normal variation of the blood pressure during respiration (i.e. the blood pressure falls during inspiration; if this fall is greater than 10 mmHg this is abnormal).

51

Jugular venous pressure

Look for:

- Kussmaul's sign—jugular venous pressure (JVP) increases with inspiration (normally, it falls), as seen in cases where pericardial effusion leads to cardiac tamponade.
- Friedreich's sign—a rapid collapse of the JVP during diastole seen in aortic regurgitation.

The JVP may be elevated due to cardiac failure.

Praecordium

Look for scars of previous valve replacement (prosthetic valves are more prone to infective endocarditis). The scar used in these operations is the median sternotomy scar. Do not forget the mitral valvotomy scar under the left breast. Closed mitral valvotomy has been superseded by mitral valvuloplasty, which is undertaken via the femoral artery, but there are still patients who have had closed mitral valvotomy to treat mitral stenosis in the past and these are also vulnerable to infective endocarditis.

Listen for:

- Murmurs, especially those of valvular incompetance caused by infective endocarditis.
- Prosthetic valve sounds.
- Pericardial rub—this may be heard in patients who have pericarditis and has been described as the squeak of new leather. It is best heard with the diaphragm of the stethoscope and can be distinguished from a heart murmur because its timing with the heart cycle often varies from beat to beat and may appear and disappear from one day to the next.

Respiratory system

Examine carefully for signs of infection such as bronchial breathing, a pleural rub, or pleural effusion.

Gastrointestinal system

Possible findings include:

- Splenomegaly, which is an important finding because it is a sign of infective endocarditis.
- Hepatomegaly, which may be found as a consequence of cardiac failure or of viral infection (e.g. infectious mononucleosis).

Skin

Infective endocarditis and many viral infections may be associated with a rash.

INVESTIGATION OF PATIENTS WHO HAVE A FEVER ASSOCIATED WITH A CARDIAC SYMPTOM OR SIGN

Blood tests

Blood cultures

This is the most important diagnostic test in infective endocarditis.

At least three sets of blood cultures should be taken, if possible 1 hour apart, from different sites before commencing antibiotics. This enables isolation of the causative organism in over 98% of cases of bacterial endocarditis. Therapy is often started immediately after this and can then be modified when the blood culture results are available.

Full blood count

A full blood count may reveal:

- Anaemia of chronic disease, which is commonly seen in patients who have infective endocarditis.
- A leucocytosis, which is an indicator of infection or inflammation.
- Thrombocytopenia, which may accompany disseminated intravascular coagulopathy in cases of severe sepsis.

Other blood tests

These include:

- Antistreptolysin O titres, which may be useful in cases of rheumatic fever.
- Monospot test if Epstein–Barr virus infection is suspected as a possible cause of viral myocarditis.
- Clotting screen because clotting may be deranged in cases of sepsis associated with disseminated intravascular coagulation.
- Renal function tests, which may be abnormal in infective endocarditis because the associated vasculitis may involve the kidneys causing glomerulonephritis. Autoimmune disease may also cause renal dysfunction and is a cause of pericarditis and myocarditis.
- Liver function tests, which are abnormal in many viral infections.
- Erythrocyte sedimentation rate and C-reactive protein measurements because these inflammatory markers are a sensitive indicator of the presence of infection or inflammation. They are also invaluable as markers of the response to treatment. Because C-reactive

protein has a short half-life (approximately 8 hours) it is often a more sensitive marker of disease activity than the erythrocyte sedimentation rate.

- Viral titres, which are taken in the acute and convalescent phase of the illness and may reveal the cause of pericarditis or myocarditis. If viral illness is suspected throat swabs and faecal culture are also appropriate investigations to isolate the organism.

Urinalysis

No examination of a cardiovascular patient is complete without dipstick of the urine to look for microscopic haematuria. This is an extremely sensitive test for infective endocarditis and must not be forgotton. Urine microscopy almost always reveals red blood cells in infective endocarditis. Proteinuria may also be a finding.

Electrocardiography

In patients who have pericarditis the ECG may show characteristic ST segment elevation. This differs from that seen in myocardial infarction because it is:

- Concave.
- Present in all leads.
- Associated with upright T waves.

Eventually with time the ST segments may flatten or invert, but unlike infarction there is no loss of R wave height.

Myocarditis may be associated with atrial arrhythmias or interventricular conduction defects. Rarely complete heart block may occur.

Chest radiography

This may reveal an underlying cause of cardiac disease:

- Pneumonia—a possible cause of atrial fibrillation.
- Lung tumour—may invade the pericardium causing pericardial effusion.
- Cardiac failure—an enlarged cardiac shadow and pulmonary oedema may be seen in patients who have valve disease or myocarditis.
- A globular heart shadow—characteristic of a pericardial effusion.
- Calcified heart valves—may be visible in a patient who has a history of rheumatic fever.

Transthoracic echocardiography

Transthoracic echocardiography is a very useful investigation in the patient who has fever and a cardiac symptom or sign:

- Left ventricular function can be accurately assessed—in myocarditis this is found to be globally reduced (in patients who have left ventricular failure due to ischaemic heart disease the left ventricle often shows regional dysfunction according to the site of the vascular lesion).
- Valve lesions may be identified and in cases of infective endocarditis the vegetations may be visualized on the valve leaflets. It is important to remember, however, that infective endocarditis cannot be excluded by the absence of vegetations on echocardiography. This investigation is by no means 100% sensitive and blood cultures remain the most important investigation for this condition.

Transoesophageal echocardiography

Transoesophageal echocardiography is more sensitive than transthoracic echocardiography because the resolution is much better. It allows a more detailed examination to be made and is especially useful in cases where transthoracic echocardiography does not provide adequate imaging, for example:

- Prosthetic heart valves—the acoustic shadows cast by these make imaging with transthoracic echocardiography very difficult.
- Localization of vegetations—transoesophageal echocardiography will visualize vegetations in many cases of infective endocarditis.

Pericardiocentesis

This may be appropriate if a pericardial effusion is found at echocardiography.

The procedure is performed by an experienced operator and uses echocardiography as a guide for positioning of a catheter in the pericardial space. An ECG lead is often attached to the needle when attempting to enter the pericardium and will show an injury current (with ST elevation) if the myocardium is touched so enabling myocardial puncture to be avoided.

Pericardiocentesis may be:

- Therapeutic—if it relieves cardiac tamponade.
- Diagnostic—if the pericardial fluid can be cultured to reveal an infective organism.

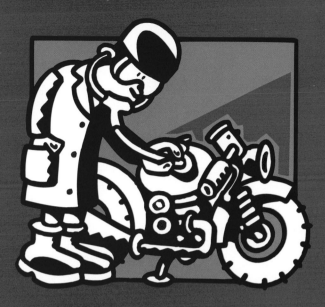

HISTORY, EXAMINATION, AND COMMON INVESTIGATIONS

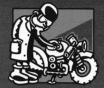

9. History

AIM OF HISTORY TAKING

The aim of history taking is to observe the following points:
- Highlight important symptoms and present them in a clear and logical manner.
- Obtain information about the severity of the symptoms and therefore of the underlying disease.
- Ask questions relevant to suspected diseases and so narrow the list of suspected differential diagnoses.
- Evaluate to what extent the individual's lifestyle has been affected by or has contributed to the underlying disease.

PRESENTING COMPLAINT

The presenting complaint will usually be one of the following:
- Chest pain.
- Dyspnoea.
- Syncope or dizziness.
- Ankle swelling.
- Palpitations.

It may be an incidental finding of a murmur or hypertension.

Chest pain

Ascertain the following points as you would for any type of pain:
- Nature of the pain (e.g. sharp, dull, heavy, burning).
- Site and radiation of the pain.
- Exacerbating and relieving factors.
- Duration of the problem—is it getting worse?
- Associated features (Fig. 9.1).

Angina means 'choking'. Patients will often deny chest pain but will describe a squeezing or crushing sensation instead.

Dyspnoea

This is an uncomfortable awareness of one's breathing. Ascertain the following:
- Precipitating factors.
- Duration of the problem—is it getting worse?
- Associated features such as chest pain, palpitations, sweating, cough or haemoptysis (Fig. 9.2)

Features of different types of chest pain					
Cause	Angina pectoris	Pericarditis	Pulmonary embolus or pneumonia	Oesophagitis or oesophageal spasm	Cervical spondylosis
Location	retrosternal	central or left-sided	anywhere in chest	epigastric or retrosternal	central or lateral
Nature	pressure or dull ache	sharp	sharp	dull or burning	aching or sharp
Radiation	left arm, neck, or jaw	no	no	neck	arms
Exacerbating factors	exertion, cold weather, stress	recumbent position, deep inspiration	deep inspiration, coughing	recumbent position, presence or lack of food	movement
Relieving features	rest, GTN spray, oxygen mask	sitting forward	stopping breathing	food or antacids, GTN spray	weather, position in bed
Associated features	shortness of breath, sweating, nausea, palpitations	shortness of breath, sweating, palpitations, fever	shortness of breath, haemoptysis, cough, fever	sweating, nausea	dizziness, pain in neck or shoulder

Fig. 9.1 Features of different types of chest pain. (GTN, glyceryl trinitrate.)

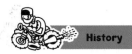

Features of the conditions causing dyspnoea		
System involved	Disease	Features of dyspnoea
cardiovascular	pulmonary oedema	may be acute or chronic, exacerbated by exertion or lying flat (orthopnoea and PND), associated with sweating (and cough with pink frothy sputum),
	ischaemic heart disease	exacerbated by exertion or stress, relieved by rest, associated with sweating and angina
respiratory	COAD	chronic onset, exacerbated by exertion and respiratory infections, may be associated with cough and sputum, always associated with history of smoking
	interstitial lung disease	chronic onset, no real exacerbating or relieving factors, may have history of exposure to occupational dusts or allergens
	pulmonary embolus	acute onset, associated with pleuritic chest pain and haemoptysis
	pneumothorax	acute onset, pleuritic chest pain
	pneumonia and neoplasms of the lung	associated with pleuritic pain
other	pregnancy	gradual progression due to splinting of diaphragm or anaemia
	obesity	gradual progression due to effort of moving and chest wall restriction
	anaemia	history of blood loss, peptic ulcer, operations, etc

Fig. 9.2 Features of conditions causing dyspnoea. (COAD, chronic obstructive airways disease; PND, paroxysmal nocturnal dyspnoea.)

Paroxysmal nocturnal dyspnoea may be the first feature of pulmonary oedema. This occurs when fluid accumulates in the lungs when the patient lies flat during sleep. When awake, the respiratory centres are very sensitive and register oedema early with dyspnoea; during sleep sensory awareness is depressed, allowing pulmonary oedema to accumulate. The patient is therefore woken by a severe sensation of breathlessness, which is extremely frightening and is relieved by sitting or standing up.

Ask about the following:
- Speed of onset.
- Precipitating events.
- Nature of the recovery period.

Cardiac syncope often occurs with no warning and is associated with rapid and complete recovery. Be careful therefore because the patient will usually be well when you take the history despite having a potentially life-threatening condition.

Syncope

This is a loss of consciousness due to inadequate perfusion of the brain. The differential diagnosis is given in Fig. 9.3.

Palpitations

Ask the following questions:
- Can you describe the palpitations?—ask the patient to tap them out.
- Are there any precipitating or relieving factors?
- How long do they last and how frequent are they?

Differential diagnosis of syncope			
Cause	Speed of onset	Precipitating events	Nature of recovery
Stokes–Adams attack (transient asystole; result from cerebral hypoxia occurring during prolonged asystole)	sudden—patient feels entirely well immediately before syncope	often none	rapid, often with no sequelae
tachycardia—VT or very rapid SVT	sudden	often none	rapid
AS and HOCM	sudden	exertion, sometimes no warning	rapid
vasovagal syncope	preceded by dizziness, rapid	sudden pain, emotion, micturition	patient often feels nauseated or vomits
orthostatic hypotension	rapid onset after standing	standing up suddenly, prolonged standing, use of antihypertensive or antianginal agents	may feel nauseated
carotid sinus hypersensitivity	dizziness or no warning	movement of the head	may feel nauseated
neurological (may be associated with convulsions during the period of unconsciousness)—epileptiform seizure or cerebrovascular event	may have classical aura or focal neurological signs, rapid onset	often none (certain types of flashing lights or alcohol withdrawal may precipitate epilepsy)	often drowsy, may have residual neurological deficit
pulmonary embolus	chest pain, dyspnoea, or no warning	none (but ask about recent travel, hospitalization, etc.)	may have dyspnoea or pleuritic chest pain
hypoglycaemia (may be associated with convulsions during the period of unconsciousness)	slower onset, nausea, sweating, tremor	exercise, insulin therapy, missing meals	often drowsy

Fig. 9.3 Differential diagnosis of syncope. (AS, aortic stenosis; HOCM, hypertrophic obstructive cardiomyopathy; SVT, supraventricular tachycardia; VT, ventricular tachycardia.)

- Are there any associated features (e.g. shortness of breath, chest pain or loss of consciousness, Fig. 9.4)?

Commonly used vagotonic manoeuvres include:
- Valsalva manoeuvre (bearing down against a closed glottis).
- Carotid sinus massage—remember only one side at a time! and listen for carotid bruits beforehand.
- Painful stimuli (e.g. immersing the hands into iced water or ocular pressure).
- Diving reflex (i.e. immersing the face in water).

Ankle swelling
Cardiac causes of ankle swelling include congestive cardiac failure (fluid retention caused by heart failure).

There are many causes of cardiac failure. Causes of left heart failure include:
- Ischaemic heart disease.
- Hypertension.

- Mitral and aortic valve disease.
- Cardiomyopathies.

Causes of right heart failure include:
- Secondary to left heart failure (congestive cardiac failure).
- Chronic lung disease (cor pulmonale).
- Pulmonary embolism.
- Tricuspid and pulmonary valve disease.
- Mitral valve disease with pulmonary hypertension.
- Right ventricular infarct.
- Primary pulmonary hypertension.

From the above list it can be seen that a history encompassing all aspects of cardiac disease needs to be taken to identify the possible causes of ankle swelling.

Ankle swelling secondary to cardiac causes is classically worse later in the day after the patient has been walking around. The hydrostatic pressure in the small blood vessels is greater when the legs are held

Causes of palpitations		
Rhythm	Precipitating factors	Relieving factors
sinus tachycardia	anxiety, exertion, thyrotoxicosis, anaemia	rest or specific treatment of underlying condition
atrial fibrillation	ischaemia, thyrotoxicosis, hypertensive heart disease, mitral valve disease, ischaemia, alcoholic heart disease, pulmonary sepsis or embolism, idiopathic	antiarrhythmic agents or treatment of the underlying disorder
atrial flutter	thyrotoxicosis, sepsis, alcohol, caffeine, pulmonary embolus, idiopathic	antiarrhythmic agents or treatment of the underlying cause
AV and AV nodal re-entry tachycardias	caffeine, emotion, alcohol, or no obvious cause	vasovagal stimulation, ablation of re-entry pathway or anti-arrhythmic drugs
VT	ischaemia, ventricular dysplasia	antiarrhythmic agents, treatment of the underlying cause or ablation of focus of arrhythmia
bradyarrhythmias (AV nodal block or sinus node disease)	often none (overtreatment of tachycardia with antiarrhythmic agents)	stop antiarrhythmic agent or insert permanent pacemaker

Fig. 9.4 Causes of palpitations. (AV, atrioventricular; VT, ventricular tachycardia.)

vertical, so increasing the accumulation of fluid in the interstitial spaces. At night, however, the legs are raised, reducing intravascular pressure and allowing flow of fluid back into the venules with reduction of the oedema by morning.

Non-cardiac causes of ankle swelling include:
- Renal—due to proteinuria.
- Hepatic—due to low serum albumin.
- Protein malnutrition—due to low serum albumin.
- Pulmonary due to hypercapnia and hypoxia in COAD.

SYSTEMS REVIEW

It is very important to learn the skill of taking a rapid, but detailed systems review. This part of the history consists of direct questions covering the important symptoms of disease affecting systems other than the one covered in the presenting complaint. Learn the questions by heart so that you automatically ask them every time you take a history (note that this is only time consuming if the doctor has trouble remembering the questions to ask).

Respiratory system
Cough
Cough may suggest the presence of infection, a common cause of arrhythmias. Cough is also a symptom of cardiac failure.

Haemoptysis
Haemoptysis is a feature of pulmonary embolism, pulmonary oedema (sputum may be pink and frothy), pulmonary hypertension secondary to mitral valve disease, and pulmonary infection.

Wheeze
This is classically seen in asthmatics (remember that asthmatics cannot take β-blockers), but is also a feature of cardiac asthma as a sign of pulmonary oedema. Patients who have chronic obstructive airways disease may complain of wheeze; these patients have often been heavy smokers and are therefore at risk of cardiac disease.

Gastrointestinal system
Appetite
Appetite is often reduced in cardiac failure because patients are too breathless to eat; this and other factors lead to cardiac cachexia.

Weight loss or gain
Oedema can cause marked weight gain. Severe cardiac failure or infective endocarditis can cause weight loss.

Nausea and vomiting
Nausea and vomiting often complicates an acute myocardial infarction, vasovagal syncope, and drug toxicity (e.g. digoxin toxicity).

Indigestion
This may be confused for ischaemic cardiac pain and vice versa.

Diarrhoea and constipation
Diarrhoea may lead to electrolyte imbalance affecting cardiac rhythm or may be a sign of viral illness leading to myocarditis or pericarditis.

Central nervous system
Headache
Headache may be a side effect of cardiac drugs (e.g. nitrates, calcium channel blockers).

Weakness, sensory loss, visual or speech disturbance
These signs may suggest thromboembolic disease, which may complicate atrial fibrillation or may alter the decision to give thrombolysis to a patient who has acute myocardial infarction.

Skin and joints
Rashes
Rashes are an important sign in the patient who has infective endocarditis or a possible drug side effect. They are also seen in many viral illnesses and autoimmune disease.

Joint pain
Joint pain can occur in infective endocarditis, viral disease, rheumatic fever, and autoimmune disease. A history of arthritis will affect the decision to undertake an exercise tolerance test to diagnose angina.

Genitourinary system
Proteinuria
This suggests a renal cause of oedema.

Haematuria
Macroscopic haematuria is sometimes seen in infective endocarditis.

Frequency, hesitancy, nocturia, and terminal dribbling
Symptoms of prostatism are common in middle-aged male patients who have heart disease and may affect their compliance with diuretic therapy.

Impotence and failure of ejaculation
These symptoms can be caused by β-blockers and are also quite common in diabetics and arteriopaths, two groups of patients commonly attending cardiology clinics and being treated in coronary care units.

Past medical history
For any patient the past medical history should include all previous illnesses and operations and the dates when they occurred. In particular, in cardiac patients emphasis should be placed on the following aspects of the past medical history:

- Risk factors for ischaemic heart disease—smoking, diabetes mellitus, hypercholesterolaemia, hypertension or family history—it may be easier to ask about this along with the other risk factors rather than in the family history section of the history.
- History of rheumatic fever.
- History of recent dental work—an important cause of infective endocarditis (others include recent invasive procedures such as upper gastrointestinal endoscopy, colonoscopy, or bladder catheterization).

Drug history
For all patients this should include all regular medications with details of doses and times. In addition, in the cardiac patient, attention should be paid to the following features:

- Any previous history of thrombolysis, in particular the administration of streptokinase because this should not be administered again within 2 years of the last dose (some centres now never administer streptokinase to a patient who has received it before preferring to use recombinant tissue plasminogen activator instead). This is because it is thought that antibodies develop to the bacterial antigens in streptokinase so rendering it less effective when administered for a second time because the drug is bound by antibodies and neutralized.
- Nitrates should be taken in such a way as to allow for a drug-free period; therefore if a twice daily nitrate is being used it is important to establish that it is not being taken at 12-hourly intervals. For example isosorbide mononitrate should be taken at 8 a.m. and 2 p.m. so that drug levels fall to very low levels overnight.
- Drugs that have cardiac effects (e.g. antidepressants, antiasthmatics).

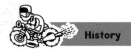

Heart conditions that have a genetic component		
Disorder	Inheritance	Cardiac complications
familial hypercholesterolaemia	AR	premature ischaemic heart disease
HOCM	AD	sudden death, arrhythmias
Marfan syndrome	AD	aortic dissection, mitral valve prolapse or incompetence
haemochromatosis	AR	cardiomyopathy
Romano–Ward, Jervell, Lange–Nielsen syndromes	AR	long QT syndrome, may lead to sudden death due to ventricular arrhythmias
homocystinuria	AR	premature ischaemic heart disease, recurrent venous thrombosis

Fig. 9.5 Heart conditions that have a genetic component. (AD, autosomal dominant; AR, autosomal recessive; HOCM, hypertrophic obstructive cardiomyopathy.)

ALLERGIES

All drug allergies should be carefully documented with information on the precise effects noted.

FAMILY HISTORY

Ischaemic heart disease is recognized as having a genetic component and this should have been ascertained earlier in the history.

In addition to this other cardiac conditions have a genetic component (Fig. 9.5).

SOCIAL HISTORY

The social history aims to identify any areas in the patient's lifestyle that may contribute to or be affected by his or her disease:

- Occupation—always ask about the patient's occupation. In cardiac patients this is particularly important because a history of ischaemic heart disease for example may result in the loss of a heavy goods vehicle licence. There are many other similar situations where a patient may not be able to continue work and these need to be identified.
- Smoking—a recognized risk factor in cardiovascular disease.
- Use of illegal drugs—intravenous drug abuse is associated with a high risk of infective endocarditis. The organisms involved are unusual (e.g. *Staphylococcus aureus, Candida albicans,* Gram-negative organisms, and anaerobes). Cocaine abuse is associated with coronary artery spasm and increased myocardial oxygen demand resulting in some cases in myocardial ischaemia and infarction. Long-term use of cocaine may result in dilated cardiomyopathy.
- Alcohol intake—heavy alcohol consumption has many cardiac effects (Fig. 9.6). Alcohol is a potent myocardial depressant when taken in excess over a long period.

Cardiovascular effects of heavy alcohol consumption	
Cardiovascular effect	**Comments**
cardiomyopathy	alcohol is the second most common cause of dilated cardiomyopathy in developed countries (the first most common being ischaemic heart disease) due to a direct toxic effect of alcohol on the myocardium and also due to a nutritional deficiency of thiamine, which often accompanies alcohol excess and may lead to beriberi; dilated cardiomyopathy is most commonly seen in men aged 35–55 years of age who have been drinking heavily for over 10 years
arrhythmias	most commonly atrial arrhythmias (e.g. atrial fibrillation, but also ventricular arrhythmias)
sudden death	due to ventricular arrhythmias
hypertension	alcohol is an independent risk factor for hypertension, possibly due to stimulation of the sympathetic nervous system
coronary artery disease	in small quantities alcohol has a protective effect on IHD, but heavy alcohol intake is associated with an increased risk of IHD

Fig. 9.6 Cardiovascular effects of heavy alcohol consumption. (IHD, ischaemic heart disease.)

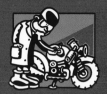

10. Examination

This chapter provides information on how to examine the cardiovascular system. The method of examination remains the same whether you are sitting for finals or for the membership examination so you should learn it properly once and for all. Remember cardiovascular cases are among the most popular used in short-case examinations.

HOW TO BEGIN THE EXAMINATION

Always start by introducing yourself and gently shaking hands (many elderly patients have painful arthritic joints—never make the patient wince when you shake hands with them). Ask the patient if you can examine his or her chest and heart.

Position the patient correctly. The patient should remove all clothing from the waist upward—it is acceptable for a female patient to cover her breasts when you are not observing or examining the praecordium.

The patient should be sitting comfortably against the pillows with his or her back at 45 degrees with the head supported so that the neck muscles are relaxed—the only two circumstances when you may deviate from this position are:

- If the patient has such bad pulmonary oedema that he or she needs to sit bolt upright.
- If the jugular venous pressure (JVP) is not raised, a more recumbent position will fill the jugular vein and allow examination of the venous pressure waveform.

OBSERVATION

As soon as you see the patient and during your introductions you should be observing the patient and his or her surroundings. Once the patient has been positioned expose the chest, step to the end of the bed, and observe for a few seconds.

Observation is an art and you will be surprised how much information you can obtain and remember after only a few seconds. In many cases this part of the examination provides valuable clues about the diagnosis. The secret to this is knowing what to look for.

Look at the patient's face for the following signs:
- Breathlessness, central cyanosis.
- Malar flush of mitral stenosis.
- Corneal arcus or xanthelasma—suggestive of hypercholesterolaemia.
- Any signs of congenital abnormality such as the classical appearance of Down syndrome (endocardial cushion defects) or Turner's syndrome (coarctation and aortic stenosis).

Look at the neck and praecordium:
- Visible pulsation in the neck may be due to a high-volume carotid pulse or giant 'v' waves in the JVP (the JVP usually has a double pulsation).
- Scars and visible pulsation on the chest (it is important to have a working knowledge of the common scars seen (Fig. 10.1) and the apex beat may be visible.

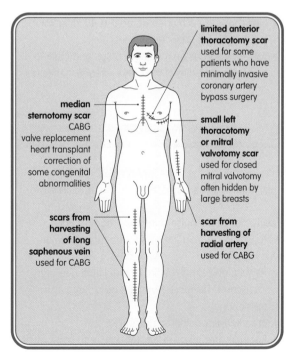

Fig. 10.1 Common scars related to cardiac surgery. Note that a larger left lateral thoracotomy is used for correction of coarction and patent ductus arteriosus. (CABG, coronary artery bypass grafting.)

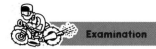

Look for peripheral oedema if the patient's feet are visible.

Look at the patient's surroundings:
- Are there intravenous infusions?—if so look at what they contain—high-dose intravenous antibiotics may suggest infective endocarditis.
- Is the patient on oxygen?—suggests heart failure or lung disease.
- Are there any diabetic drinks or food?—diabetics have a high incidence of ischaemic heart disease.

All this can be done very rapidly—it tends to irritate examiners if you spend more than about 15–30 s on observation.

Causes of clubbing	
System involved	Pathology
respiratory	carcinoma of the lung (especially squamous cell), suppurative lung conditions (e.g. lung abscess, empyema, bronchiectasis), fibrosing alveolitis
cardiovascular	cyanotic heart disease, infective endocarditis (takes several weeks for clubbing to develop)
gastrointestinal	inflammatory bowel disease, cirrhosis

Fig. 10.2 Causes of clubbing.

EXAMINATION OF THE HANDS

Pick up the patient's right hand gently (alternatively you can ask the patient to lift both hands and look at them one after the other so avoiding the risk of causing any pain). Look for the following:
- Peripheral cyanosis and cold peripheries —suggests peripheral vascular disease or poor cardiac output.
- Nail changes such as clubbing (Fig. 10.2), splinter haemorrhages, nicotine staining.
- Janeway lesions on the finger pulps and Osler's nodes on the palm of the hand—suggest infective endocarditis.

EXAMINATION OF THE PULSE

After examining the pulse you should be able to comment on three things: rate, rhythm and character.

Feel for the radial pulse and time it against your watch for 15–30 s. At the same time make note of whether it is:
- Regular and sinus rhythm or atrial flutter/re-entry tachycardia if rapid—note that atrial flutter may be slow.
- Irregularly irregular—atrial fibrillation.
- Regularly irregular—Wenckebach heart block gives this rhythm because the PR interval progressively lengthens and finally a beat is dropped—you are very unlikely to be asked to diagnose Wenckebach rhythm by feeling the pulse.

Don't get confused by occasional ectopic beats, which make the pulse seem irregularly irregular for a short time. In these patients it is important to feel the pulse for at least 15 s because you will notice that the basic rhythm is sinus.

The character of the pulse is usually best assessed at the carotid pulse, but you may notice a slow rising pulse at the radial pulse (Fig. 10.3).

A collapsing pulse can usually be felt by gently lifting the patient's arm and feeling the pulse with the fingers laid across it. The impulse is felt as it hits the examiner's finger and then rapidly declines.

Finally check briefly for radioradial delay by feeling both radial pulses together. This may result from coarctation of the aorta (proximal to the left subclavian artery) or unilateral subclavian artery stenosis.

TAKE THE BLOOD PRESSURE

Always ask whether you can take the blood pressure yourself and be sure that you know how to do this properly.

Strictly speaking, the blood pressure should be measured in both arms, but examiners will probably not ask you to do this unless it is likely to be abnormal (suggesting coarctation of the aorta).

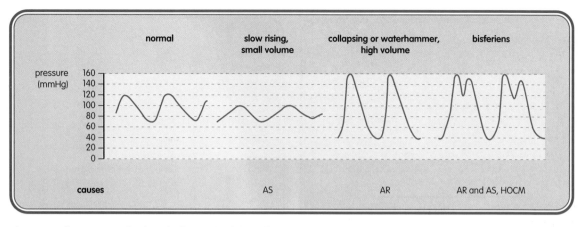

Fig. 10.3 Different types of pulse. The first peak of the bisferiens pulse is caused by left ventricular contraction (the percussion wave); the second peak is the tidal wave due to recoil of the vascular bed. (AR, aortic regurgitation; AS, aortic stenosis; HOCM, hypertrophic obstructive cardiomyopathy.)

Postural hypotension describes a drop in blood pressure in a person who has been standing for more than 2 min of more than 20 mmHg compared with when he or she is lying down.

Pulsus paradoxus describes an exaggeration of the normal (not actually a paradox) blood pressure on inspiration (>10 mmHg less than on expiration)—causes are cardiac tamponade, constrictive pericarditis, severe asthma.

EXAMINATION OF THE FACE

Keep this brief because you should have observed the face earlier.

Additional information can be obtained by looking at the conjunctivae. The presence of conjunctival haemorrhages suggests infective endocarditis, the presence of conjunctival pallor suggests anaemia.

Look briefly in the mouth for:
• Nicotine staining of the teeth—seen in heavy smokers.
• Central cyanosis.

EXAMINATION OF THE JUGULAR VENOUS PRESSURE

This is sometimes difficult so make things easier by ensuring the patient is in the correct position (at 45 degrees with the head supported and the neck muscles relaxed).

The internal jugular vein is used because it has no valves and is not subject to as much muscular compression as the external jugular vein. The JVP gives an indication of the right atrial pressure (Fig. 10.4). The normal JVP is less than 3 cmH$_2$O (measured as the vertical distance above the angle of Louis). This rests at the level of the clavicle so the normal JVP waveform is not usually visible or, if it is seen, the pulsation is just above the clavicle. It can be visualized by lying the patient flat. In sinus rhythm, there are two waves:
• 'a' just preceding the carotid pulse—this is absent in atrial systole.
• 'v', which is accentuated in tricuspid regurgitation.

Occasional 'cannon' waves are seen in heart block when the right atrium contracts against a closed tricuspid valve.

The differences between the JVP and carotid pulse are highlighted in Fig. 10.5.

Kussmaul's sign

Normally the JVP falls with inspiration because the pressure in the thoracic cavity is negative. In constrictive

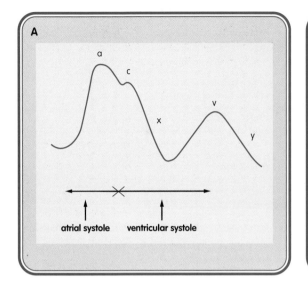

Fig. 10.4 (A) Jugular venous pressure (JVP) waveform. **(B)** Causes of the waves and descents in the JVP.

B	Causes of waves and descents in the JVP
Wave or descent	**Cause**
a wave	right atrial systole, which results in venous distension
c wave	increasing right ventricular pressure just before the tricuspid valve closes producing an interruption in the x descent
x descent	atrial relaxation and pulling down of the base of the atrium caused by right ventricular contraction
v wave	right atrial filling during right ventricular systole
y descent	fall in right atrial pressure as the tricuspid valve opens

Differences between the JVP and carotid pulse		
Feature	**JVP**	**Carotid pulse**
character of pulse	double pulsation: a wave occurs at end of diastole, v wave with systole	single systolic pulse
potential for obliteration	can be obliterated by pressing on vein just above the clavicle	cannot be obliterated
effect of position	if the patient sits upright it falls	no effect
effect of pressure on the liver or abdomen	rises (the hepatojugular reflex)	no effect
palpable pulsation	usually not palpable	palpable

Fig. 10.5 Differences between the jugular venous pressure (JVP) and carotid pulse.

pericarditis or cardiac tamponade the JVP increases with inspiration this is known as Kussmaul's sign.

EXAMINATION OF THE PRAECORDIUM

Palpation
The following sequence of palpation should be observed:
- Palpate the apex beat, defined as the lowest and most lateral point at which the cardiac impulse can be felt. Always start palpating in the axilla and move anteriorly until you feel the apex beat. If you start

palpating anteriorly it is possible to miss a grossly displaced apex. Define the character of the apex beat (Fig. 10.6).
- Palpate the left lower sternal edge to feel for a right ventricular heave (a sign of pulmonary hypertension or pulmonary stenosis)—use the flat of the hand pressing firmly to feel this.
- Palpate the second left intercostal space where a palpable pulmonary component of the second heart sound (P_2) may be felt (a sign of pulmonary hypertension). This is felt with the fingertips.
- Palpate the second right intercostal space where a palpable thrill of aortic stenosis may be felt—this is also felt with the fingertips.

Percussion

Percussion of the heart is rarely performed and can be excluded from the routine examination. The area of cardiac dullness is affected by lung conditions (e.g. emphysema). However, an increased area of dullness indicates cardiac enlargement or pericardial effusion. This is useful if the apex beat is not palpable.

Causes of different types of apex beat	
Character	Causes
tapping	MS
thrusting	MR, AR
heaving	AS
diffuse (the normal apex beat should be discrete and localized to an area no bigger than a 10-pence piece)	left ventricular failure, cardiomyopathy
double	HOCM, left ventricular aneurysm

Fig. 10.6 Causes of different types of apex beat. (AR, aortic regurgitation; AS, aortic stenosis; HOCM, hypertrophic obstructive cardiomyopathy; MR, mitral regurgitation; MS, mitral stenosis.)

Auscultation

When listening to the heart every murmur should be systematically excluded. You should at all times be able to explain exactly which sounds you are expecting to hear at any stage during auscultation.

Learn a systematic approach, not necessarily the one described in this chapter, but always listen to the heart in the same way.

Knowing when systole and diastole are is fundamental. Know this at all times during auscultation by keeping a finger or thumb on the carotid pulse.

The order for auscultation is as follows:

- Using the diaphragm of the stethoscope listen quickly at the mitral, tricuspid, pulmonary, and aortic areas in that order—you should already know where these are; if not then learn it now (Fig 10.7). This enables

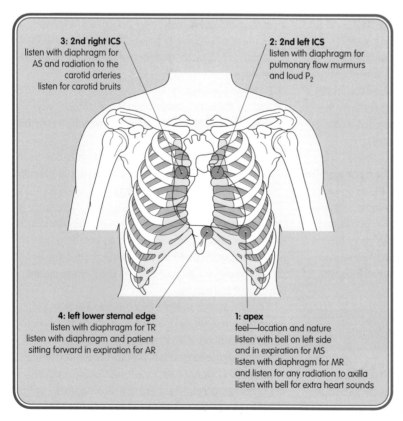

Fig. 10.7 Sequence of auscultation of the heart. (AR, aortic regurgitation; AS, aortic stenosis; ICS, intercostal space; MR, mitral regurgitation; MS, mitral stenosis; TR, tricuspid regurgitation.)

3: 2nd right ICS
listen with diaphragm for AS and radiation to the carotid arteries
listen for carotid bruits

2: 2nd left ICS
listen with diaphragm for pulmonary flow murmurs and loud P_2

4: left lower sternal edge
listen with diaphragm for TR
listen with diaphragm and patient sitting forward in expiration for AR

1: apex
feel—location and nature
listen with bell on left side and in expiration for MS
listen with diaphragm for MR and listen for any radiation to axilla
listen with bell for extra heart sounds

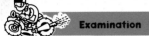

you to hear any loud murmurs and possibly begin to approach the diagnosis.

- Listen at the apex: first with the bell of the stethoscope to hear any extra heart sounds (i.e. third and fourth heart sounds); listen for mitral stenosis by asking the patient to lie on his or her left side and breathe out fully. Again the bell of the stethoscope should be used for this. Listen for mitral regurgitation at the apex with the diaphragm of the stethoscope. If a pansystolic murmur is heard listen at the axilla for radiation of the murmur.

> **You cannot say that mitral stenosis has been excluded unless you have listened with the bell of the stethoscope at the apex with the patient lying on his or her left side in full expiration.**

- Listen at the pulmonary area—using the diaphragm to hear a pulmonary flow murmur and loud P_2 if present. Both are accentuated in inspiration.
- Listen in the aortic area for the ejection systolic murmur of aortic stenosis using the diaphragm. This murmur is usually loud, but if there is any doubt ask the patient to exhale, because left-sided murmurs are loudest in expiration. Take this opportunity to listen over the carotid arteries for radiation of an aortic stenotic murmur if one is present or for evidence of carotid artery stenosis.
- Finally listen over the tricuspid area for a pansystolic murmur of tricuspid regurgitation or the murmur of HOCM. Then ask the patient to sit forward and listen in expiration for the murmur of aortic regurgitation (this murmur is often soft and requires accentuation by asking the patient to exhale). Both murmurs are heard best with the diaphragm of the stethoscope.

FINISHING OFF THE EXAMINATION

The rest of the examination must be completed efficiently and thoroughly with just as much care as the first part of the cardiovascular examination. The aim of

this part of the examination is to look for signs of cardiac failure and for any peripheral signs to confirm the diagnosis, which by now you may suspect:

- At this stage the patient is sitting forwards so start with auscultation of the lung bases. Listen for fine end-inspiratory crepitations and assess how far up the chest these extend (an evaluation of the severity of pulmonary oedema).
- Pleural effusions occur in heart failure and are detected by finding dullness to percussion at one or both lung bases.
- With the patient still sitting forwards check for sacral oedema by gently pressing over the sacrum for at least 10 s. Then ask the patient to sit back against the pillows
- Look for ankle oedema, again very gently, and assess how far up the leg the oedema extends (a guide to its severity). Remember oedema is often tender.

At this stage, in the short cases, it is reasonable to step back and conclude verbally by stating that you would like to go on to do the following:

- Examine the abdomen for ascites and hepatomegaly (signs of congestive cardiac failure) and for an abdominal aortic aneurysm (an expansile mass)
- Examine all peripheral pulses by palpation and listen for bruits to look for evidence of peripheral vascular disease.
- Examine the fundi.
- Look at the temperature chart for all patients who have a valve lesion to look for a fever, which may be due to infective endocarditis.
- Dipstick the patient's urine—haematuria is a very sensitive test for infective endocarditis and proteinuria is associated with renal oedema.

Obviously if you suspect that the patient has coarctation of the aorta then it is mandatory to examine the peripheral pulses and look for radiofemoral delay as part of the examination and not to just say you would like to do it at the end.

It can be seen therefore that the conclusion of the examination depends upon what you think the diagnosis may be. If in doubt do the complete cardiovascular examination until you are told to stop.

When you are not in the short case situation (if you are clerking a patient 'for real' or in the long case section of finals) always complete the whole examination.

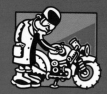

11. How to Write a Medical Clerking

There is no single correct way to write a medical clerking, but there are several incorrect ways! Remember that doctors, nurses, physiotherapists, and many other health professionals use the medical notes during the course of a patient's medical care. The notes need to last for years and your entries in them may provide valuable information to doctors looking after the patient in several years time. It is also worth remembering that the medical notes are legal documents that may one day be used as evidence in a court of law.

The basic principles when making entries into the notes are as follows

- Always write legibly—this sounds obvious, but notes are often illegible. Remember if no one else can read your entry you may as well not write anything.
- A date and time should precede every entry no matter how brief. At the end of the entry you should sign your name and, if your signature does not clearly show your name, your surname and initials should be written in capitals below it. There are no exceptions to this rule ever!
- Always be courteous to your patients and colleagues when writing in the notes. Rude or angry entries may give a certain degree of satisfaction when they are made, but only serve to make you look unprofessional when read at a later date.
- Write everything down. Every time you see a patient an entry should be made in the notes stating accurately the content and outcome of the consultation. This may sometimes seem pedantic, but most qualified doctors will be able to recall situations when careful documentation has resolved difficult situations.

DOCUMENTATION OF THE HISTORY

The history should always have the following information at the top of the first page:

- Name of patient in full plus at least one other unique identifier (e.g. date of birth or hospital number)—

loose sheets often fall out of the notes so all pages of the history should have this information so they are not replaced in the notes of another patient who has the same name.
- Date and time of entry.
- Route of admission—if the patient is being admitted to hospital it is useful to state the route by which the admission came about (i.e. via general practitioner or accident and emergency).

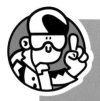

Remember, the main headings of the history are:
- Presenting complaint (PC or C/O—complains of)
- History of presenting complaint (HPC)
- Systems review (SR)
- Past medical history (PMH)
- Drug history (DH)
- Allergies
- Family history (FH)
- Social history (SH)

Presenting complaint

This should be a short list of the presenting complaint(s). There is no place in this section for any descriptions.

The purpose of the presenting complaint section is to state clearly the patient's main symptoms so that an initial differential diagnosis can be formulated. It is important that at this stage the list of differential diagnoses is large.

Examples of presenting complaints are shown in the chapter titles in the first half of this book:
- Shortness of breath.
- Palpitations (see Chapter 4).
- Collapse.
- Ankle swelling (see Chapter 5).
- Chest pain (see Chapter 1).

History of the presenting complaint

It is here that information regarding the presenting complaint is expanded. A full description of the presenting compaint(s) in turn should be noted.

It is also important in this section to ask other relevant questions pertaining to the likely organ system(s) involved. For example:

- A patient presenting with chest pain should be asked fully about the nature of the pain and should also be asked about all relevant cardiovascular and respiratory symptoms.
- In a patient who has abdominal pain a full gastrointestinal and genitourinary systems review should be included in the HPC.

Systems review

A full systems review of the other organ systems should be entered here (Fig. 11.1).

It is not necessary to document negatives unless they are particularly relevant.

Once you have memorized the questions they will become second nature and the systems review will be very quick to do. It is worth the initial time-consuming effort to do this properly; after all you will be taking histories for the rest of your career.

Past medical history

All previous illnesses and operations should be noted along with details of when they happened and if there were any complications.

Patients may be very vague about these details and you may need to speak to the relatives or the general practitioner for more information.

Drug history

All drugs taken should be documented.

Remember you cannot say you have a drug history unless the doses and times of all drugs are accurately and legibly written down.

Allergies

Not only should the drugs that the patient is allergic to be documented, but the type of reaction and when it occurred should be stated.

Fig. 11.1 Important questions to ask on systems review.

Important questions to ask on systems review	
System	Symptoms and signs to ask about
cardiovascular (CVS)	chest pain, shortness of breath, orthpnoea, paroxysmal nocturnal dyspnoea, ankle oedema, palpitations, syncope
respiratory (RS)	cough, sputum, haemoptysis, shortness of breath, wheeze
gastrointestinal (GIT)	appetite, vomiting, haematemesis, weight loss, indigestion, abdominal pain, change in bowel habit, description and frequency of stools, blood and /or mucus per rectum
genitourinary (GUS)	frequency, dysuria, hesitancy, urgency, poor stream, terminal dribbling, impotence, haematuria, menstrual cycle, menorrhagia, oligomenorrhoea, dyspareunia
neurological (CNS)	headache, photophobia, neck stiffness, visual problems, any other focal symptoms (e.g. weakness, numbness; don't forget olfactory problems), tremor, memory, loss of consciousness
other	for example muscle pain, joint pain, rashes, depression

Many patients say they are allergic to penicillin when they have only experienced some gastric discomfort while taking it. In the situation when the patient is readmitted with for example suspected meningitis this may influence whether or not a potentially life-saving dose of benzylpenicillin can be given safely.

Family history

Any diseases that have a potential genetic causation should be documented. The family member who had the disease and whether it was the cause of death should be stated.

Social history

This should include notes on the following:
- Accurate alcohol and drug intake history.
- Smoking—should be carefully documented (i.e. what is smoked, how many, for how long).

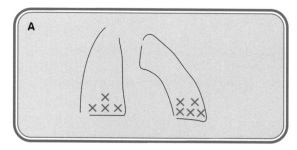

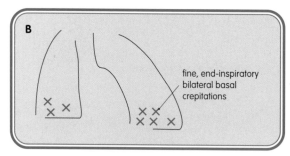

Fig. 11.2 Potential confusion caused by lack of annotation. **(A)** This diagram is usually used to represent bilateral basal crepitations secondary to pulmonary oedema. The same diagram, however, may be used to represent coarse inspiratory crepitations due to bronchiectasis. **(B)** This diagram is unequivocal and confirms the finding of pulmonary oedema.

- Occupation and possible exposure to industrial dusts or chemicals.
- If HIV infection is a possible differential diagnosis, a thorough history of possible risk factors. This may be embarrassing both for you and for the patient, but it is important not to miss a diagnosis as serious as this.

DOCUMENTATION OF THE EXAMINATION FINDINGS

There are many ways of documenting the findings on examination and it does not really matter how you do this provided a few rules are obeyed:
- The patient's name and another unique identifier are written on every sheet of paper—this should come as second nature to you.
- Any positive findings are represented in writing—diagrams can be used to aid the description, but should never be used alone to document findings because they are likely to be interpreted differently by different people (Fig. 11.2).

AT THE END OF THE CLERKING

The last section is important because it brings together all the information from the clerking. The following should be seen at the end of every clerking:
- A list of differential diagnoses with the most likely diagnosis at the top of the list.
- A list of investigations performed and to be performed—it is good practice to tick those tests that have been done already.
- A plan of action including initial drugs to be given, any intravenous fluids, physiotherapy, specific observations needed (e.g. fluid balance chart or daily weights and any consultant referrals to be made).

This reads like a long list, but you do not need to learn it. The only thing you need to remember is that if you do something that concerns a patient then write it down.

SAMPLE MEDICAL CLERKING

Abbreviations used in this sample medical clerking: D.O.B., date of birth; Hosp. No., hospital number; C/O, complaining of; HPC, history of presenting complaint; GIT, gastrointestinal tract; CNS, central nervous system; GUS, genitourinary system; PMH, past medical history; DH, drug history; GP, general practitioner; FH, family history; SH, social history; O/E, on examination; CVS, cardiovascular system; BP, blood pressure; JVP, jugular venous pressure; HS, heart sounds; S_1, first heart sound; S_2, second heart sound; P_2, pulmonary component of second heart sound; RS, respiratory system; PR, rectal examination; FBC, full blood count; U+E, urea and electrolytes; LFT, liver function tests; TFT, thyroid function tests; b.d., twice daily.

DETAILS

Mr John Smith
D.O.B. 11/06/35
Hosp. No. 345678
63-yr-old man

C/O: shortness of breath

HPC: Gradual onset of shortness of breath approximately 6 months ago.

Initially only on exertion, but breathlessness has deteriorated and now patient is breathless on minimal exertion (e.g. when dressing in the morning).

Associated features:

Orthopnoea
Ankle swelling
Cough with clear sputum and occasional flecks of blood
Palpitations—feels heart beating rapidly and irregularly from time to time with no obvious
    precipitating factors
No chest pain
No known risk factors for coronary artery disease
NB patient unaware of his cholesterol level.

Systems review

GIT: Recent loss of appetite
            No weight loss or vomiting
            No abdominal pain
            No change in bowel habit

CNS: No abnormalities on questioning
GUS: No abnormalities on questioning
PMH: Rheumatic fever when 10 years old
          Cholecystectomy 1989 no complications
DH: Frusemide 40 mg mane—started by GP last week
Allergies: None known
FH: Mother died aged 68—stroke
          Father still alive—hypertensive
SH   Never smoked
          Alcohol—approx. 10 units a week
          Retired accountant
          Married with 2 children (family fit and well)

O/E

Looks short of breath at rest. Temperature 36.5°C
No central or peripheral cyanosis.

CVS: Pulse 80, regular
          BP 120/80 mmHg
          JVP—elevated 6 cm
          Apex not displaced
          Soft low-pitched mid-diastolic murmur at apex

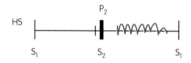

          Marked right ventricular heave and loud P_2
          Ankle oedema to knees.

RS: Respiratory rate 30 breaths/min
          Percussion and expansion normal
          Fine inspiratory bilateral basal crepitations to mid-zones

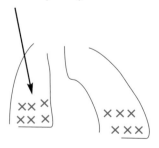

GIT: 2 cm hepatomegaly

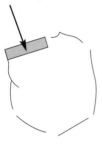

        Ascites detected

        No palpable kidneys or spleen

        PR not performed

CNS: No abnormalities detected on full neurological examination

Summary

Progressive dyspnoea in a man who has a history of rheumatic fever and clinical signs of mitral stenosis

Diagnosis

Pulmonary oedema and congestive cardiac failure secondary to rheumatic mitral stenosis

Differential diagnosis

Mitral stenosis of another aetiology

Paroxysmal atrial fibrillation leading to congestive cardiac failure

Investigations

Blood tests: FBC, U+E, LFT, TFT

Chest radiography

ECG and 24-hour ECG to rule out paroxysmal atrial fibrillation

Echocardiography

Treatment plan

Intravenous diuretics, initially frusemide 80 mg b.d.

Daily U+E to check effect of diuretics on electrolytes and renal function

Daily weights and fluid input and output chart

Fluid restriction to 1500 ml/24 hours

Referral to consultant cardiologist

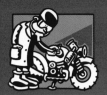

ELECTROCARDIOGRAPHY

This investigation records the electrical activity of the heart.

Lead placement
You will be expected to be able to position the electrodes correctly (Fig. 12.1) and perform an ECG by yourself so be sure to learn this before finals.

Limb leads
There are four limb leads, one attached to each extremity:
- Left arm (LA).
- Left foot (LF).
- Right arm (RA).
- Right foot (RF).

Chest leads
There are six chest leads:
- V1—4th right intercostal space.
- V2—4th left intercostal space.
- V3—between V2 and V4.
- V4—cardiac apex—you need to feel for it before placing the lead.
- V5—anterior axillary line at same level as V4
- V6—Midaxillary line at same level.

12-lead ECG
The standard 12-lead ECG is derived from information given by the ten ECG electrodes placed on the patient.

It is important to know how this information is obtained when interpreting ECG findings and also when the lead positioning is incorrect.

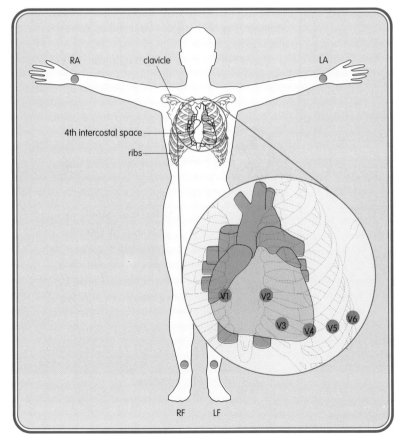

Fig. 12.1 Lead positions for electrocardiography. (LA, left arm; LF, left foot; RA, right arm; RF, right foot.)

Leads I, II, and III

These are bipolar leads and were first used by Einthoven. They record the differences in potential between pairs of limb leads:

- I records the difference in potential between LA and RA.
- II records the difference in potential between LF and RA.
- III records the difference in potential between LF and LA.

These three leads form Einthoven's triangle (Fig. 12.2).

AVR, AVL, and AVF

With regard to these leads:

- The letter V indicates that the lead is unipolar.
- The information is obtained by connecting the electrode to a central point, which is said to have zero voltage (the reference electrode).
- AVR records the difference between RA and zero.
- AVL records the difference between LA and zero.
- AVF records the difference between LF and zero.

Chest leads

The chest leads:

- Are the precordial leads V1 to V6 and are unipolar (as seen by the prefix V).
- They each record the difference between the voltage at their location and zero.

QRS axis

The normal axis is between −30 and +90 degrees (Fig. 12.3).

The most accurate way to calculate the axis (Fig. 12.4) is to take the lead in which the complex is isoelectric (i.e. the complex with equal magnitude in the positive and negative direction). Once this lead has been identified the QRS axis can be found because it is at right angles to this.

Causes of right and left axis deviation are given in Fig. 12.5.

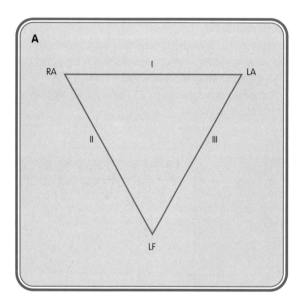

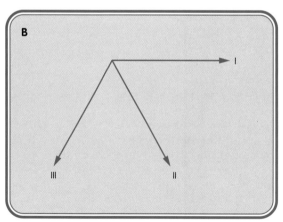

A simpler way for roughly estimating the axis is as follows:
- The normal axis is in the same direction as I and II, therefore both should be positive.
- In right axis deviation the axis swings to the right and lead I becomes negative and III more positive.
- In left axis deviation the axis swings to the left so lead III and lead II become negative and lead I remains positive.

Fig. 12.2 Leads I, II, and III. **(A)** Lead I is 0 degrees to the horizontal, II is +60 degrees to the horizontal, and lead III is +120 degrees to the horizontal—Einthoven's triangle. **(B)** Leads I, II, and III are often drawn as shown here.

Fig. 12.3 Hexaxial reference system.

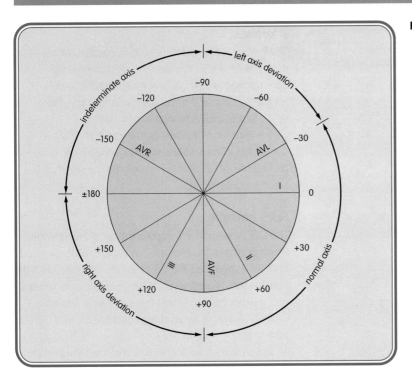

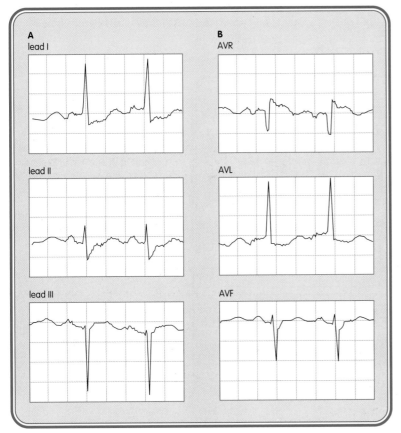

Fig. 12.4 Calculation of the axis. The QRS complex that is almost isoelectric is in lead II. Using the hexaxial reference system the two leads at right angles are –30 and +150 degrees. The axis is –30 degrees because the positive lead I excludes +150 degrees.

Causes of right and left axis deviation	
left axis deviation	LBBB, left anterior hemiblock, LVH, septum primum ASD
right axis deviation	RBBB, RVH, cor pulmonale, septum secundum ASD

Fig. 12.5 Causes of right and left axis deviation. (ASD, atrial septal defect; LBBB, left bundle branch block; LVH, left ventricular hypertrophy; RBBB, right bundle branch block; RVH, right ventricular hypertrophy.)

Paper speed

The standard ECG paper speed is 25 mm/s:
- One large square (5 mm) is 0.2 s.
- One small square (1 mm) is 0.04 s.

The rate is calculated by counting the number of large squares between each QRS and dividing into 300 (e.g. if there are five large squares the rate is 60 beats/min).

P wave

The P wave represents atrial depolarization, which originates in the SA node on the right atrium and spreads across the right and then the left atria.

The duration of the P wave is normally less than 0.12 s (three small squares)

The PR interval represents the time taken for conduction of the impulse to pass through the AV node and bundle of His. This is normally no greater than five small squares (0.2 s).

QRS complex

The QRS represents the depolarization of the ventricles, which begins at the septum. The septum is depolarized from left to right and the left and right ventricles are then depolarized. The left ventricle has a larger muscle mass and therefore more current flows across it. The left ventricle therefore exerts more influence on the ECG pattern than the right.

The maximum normal duration of the QRS is 0.12 s (three small squares) and the QRS is abnormally wide in bundle branch block (left and right bundle branch block, Chapter 18). It is also wide when the ventricles are paced (Fig. 12.6).

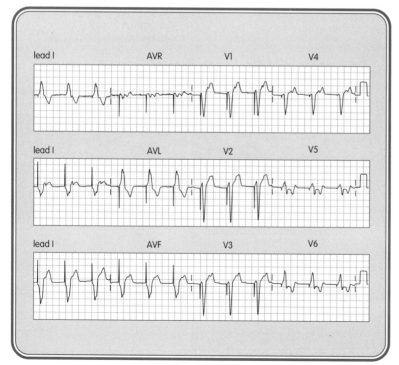

Fig. 12.6 Ventricular pacing. The sharp spikes are the artificial stimuli from the pacemaker. Each is followed by a wide QRS complex indicating the left ventricular response. Whenever the impulse is generated in one ventricle either due to a pacing wire or a ventricular ectopic focus, the QRS is widened. This mimics the electrical disturbances seen in bundle branch block because the two ventricles are not depolarized in the normal sequence.

ST segment
This segment is normally isoelectric (i.e. it shows no deflection from the baseline).

T wave
The T wave represents ventricular repolarization. Normally the only leads that show negative T waves are AVR and V1 the rest are positive. (A negative QRS should, however, be accompanied by a negative T wave.) Certain T wave abnormalities suggest particular non-cardiac disorders (Fig. 12.7).

QT interval
The QT interval extends from the beginning of the QRS complex to the end of the T wave and therefore represents time from depolarization to repolarization of the ventricles.

The duration of the QT interval is dependent upon cycle length and the corrected QT interval (QTc) is normalized (QTc = QT/square root of RR in s). The upper limit of normal is 0.39 in women and 0.44 in men.

Q waves
A Q wave is a negative deflection at the beginning of the ventricular depolarization. Small non-significant Q waves are often seen in the left-sided leads due to the depolarization of the septum from left to right. Significant Q waves:
- Are more than 0.04 s (one small square) in duration and more than 2 mm in depth.
- Occur after transmural myocardial infarction where the myocardium on one side of the heart dies.

This myocardium has no electrical activity and therefore the leads facing it are able to pick up the electrical activity from the opposite side of the heart. (The myocardium depolarizes from the inside out, therefore the opposite side of the heart depolarizes away from these leads, resulting in a negative deflection or Q wave.)

U wave
This is an abnormal wave in some patients, but can appear in the chest leads of normal ECGs. It is an upright wave that appears after the T wave (Fig. 12.8) and causes include:
- Hypokalaemia.
- Hypocalcaemia.

Reporting an ECG
You will often be asked to comment on an ECG and it is difficult to remember to include everything. This exercise should be treated like the history or the examination in that you should always follow a strict routine. After a short time this will become second nature to you.

The order of examination of an ECG is as follows:
- Name of the patient and date of the ECG.
- Rate (i.e. the number of large squares between the QRS complexes divided into 300).
- Rhythm (e.g. regular, irregular, irregularly irregular).
- Look at each part of the complex—P waves, QRS complexes, T waves, PR interval, and QRS duration —comment on these either out loud when you are starting to do this or in your head when you are more experienced, and comment on any abnormalities.

ECG abnormalities in non-cardiac disease	
Cause	ECG abnormalities
hypothermia	J waves, baseline shiver artefact, bradycardia, watch out for arrhythmias as the patient is warmed up
hyperkalaemia	tall peaked T waves, small P wave, gradual widening of the QRS, if serum potassium very high—ventricular fibrillation
hypokalaemia	decreased T wave amplitude. long QT interval, U waves
hypocalcaemia	long QT interval, U waves
hypercalcaemia	short QT interval, ST segment depression
digoxin	downsloping ST segment (reverse tick shape), T wave inversion
digoxin toxicity	AV block, atrial tachycardia with block, ventricular arrhythmias

Fig. 12.7 Electrocardiographic abnormalities in non-cardiac disease. (AV, atrioventricular.)

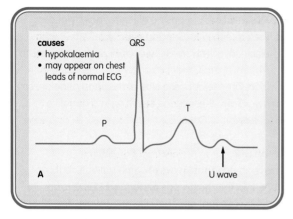

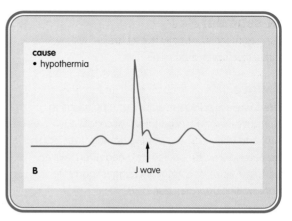

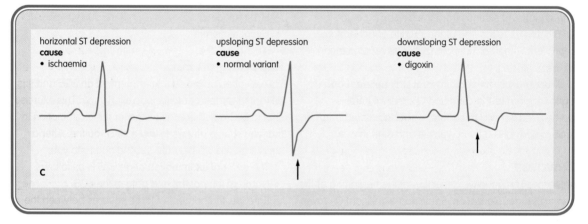

Fig. 12.8 U waves, J waves, and ST segment depression.

If there are abnormalities look to see whether they are global or territorial. Remember the territories:

- Anterior—V1–V4.
- Inferior—II, III, and AVF.
- Lateral—I, AVL, V4–V6.

When reporting an ECG:
- **Note the patient's name and date.**
- **Look at the rate and rhythm.**
- **Comment on P, QRS, and T waves (note shape and duration).**
- **Look at the distribution of changes—is it global or regional?**

Exercise electrocardiography

This investigation is important in the diagnosis of ischaemic heart disease. In addition it provides prognostic information.

Indications for exercise testing

The most common indication for exercise testing is to establish the diagnosis of ischaemic heart disease in a symptomatic patient. Other indications are as follows

- After myocardial infarction to evaluate prognosis.
- After myocardial infarction to aid rehabilitation —this gives the patient and doctor an idea of exercise capabilities.
- After angioplasty to evaluate results of treatment.
- To detect exercise-induced arrhythmias—the increased catecholamine levels and metabolic acidosis caused by exercise potentiate arrhythmias in those patients vulnerable to this. This gives an indication of prognosis and whether treatment is required or not.

Methods of exercise

The aim of the exercise test is to stress the cardiovascular system.

All exercise protocols have a warm-up period, a period of exercise with increasing grades of intensity, and a cool-down period.

The best method is treadmill exercise. Other methods such as bicycle testing are often less effective because many patients are not used to the cycling action and therefore leg fatigue often sets in before cardiovascular fatigue resulting in early termination of the test. However, bicycle testing has the advantage that the workload can be controlled and recorded in watts.

The Bruce protocol is often used in conjunction with treadmill testing. This involves 3-min stages starting with 3 min at a speed of 1.7 miles/hour and a slope of 10 degrees. Subsequent stages are at incrementally higher speeds and steeper gradients. The final stage (stage 6) is at a rate of 5.5 miles/hour and a gradient of 20 degrees.

The modified Bruce protocol is sometimes used for patients likely to have poor exercise tolerance. An additional two stages are added to the beginning of the standard Bruce protocol. Again they are 3 min in duration and at a speed of 1.7 miles/hour, but the gradient starts at 0 and increases to 5 degrees in the first and second stage, respectively.

Patient preparation

The following should be completed before testing:
- All patients should have been seen and examined by a physician to ensure there are no contraindications to testing.
- The test and its indications and risks should have been fully explained to the patient.

Certain patients are advised to stop all antihypertensive and antianginal medication before the test. The operator should be aware of patients still taking their medication because this affects the response to exercise.

Variables measured
12-lead ECG
The patient is fitted with the standard 12-lead ECG equipment. Poor electrode contact is avoided by shaving hair and gently abrading the skin with sandpaper or gauze.

Blood pressure
Normal response to exercise involves an increase in blood pressure sometimes with the systolic pressure rising up to 200 mmHg. An inadequate response or a fall in blood pressure with exercise indicates the likelihood of the following disorders:
- Coronary artery disease—the most common cause.
- Cardiomyopathy.
- Left ventricular outflow tract obstruction.
- Hypotensive medication.

Heart rate response
Heart rate normally increases with exercise. If the increase is inadequate ischaemic heart disease or sinus node disease must be suspected (also ingestion of β-blockers and calcium channel antagonists).

An excessive increase in heart rate indicates reduced cardiac reserve as in left ventricular failure or anaemia.

These variables are measured before, during, and after exercise. Measurements are stopped once all variables have returned to their pre-exercise levels.

Test end-points
The following are appropriate indications for terminating an exercise test:
- Attainment of maximal heart rate (in a modified Bruce protocol the submaximal heart rate is used, which is 85% of maximal heart rate—maximal heart rate is 220–age in years).
- Completion of all stages of the test with no untoward symptoms and without attaining maximum heart rate.

Premature termination of the exercise test is indicated if any of the following occur:
- Excessive dyspnoea or fatigue.
- Chest pain.
- Dizziness or faintness.
- Any form of arrhythmia.
- Failure of blood pressure to increase or an excessive increase in blood pressure (e.g. systolic >220 mmHg).
- Failure of heart rate to increase.
- ST segment depression greater than 1 mm.
- ST segment elevation.

Positive exercise test
The following are indications of a positive exercise test (i.e. highly suggestive of coronary artery disease):

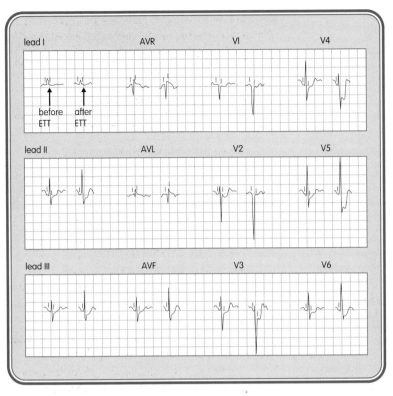

Fig. 12.9 Computer-averaged exercise ECG report showing ST depression after exercise (right-hand trace) compared with resting ECG (left-hand trace) in each of the ECG leads. There is a good tachycardia in response to exercise and the blood pressure rises to 166/84 mmHg. The ST depression is in the lateral leads V3–V6 and the inferior leads II, III, and AVF. (ETT, exercise tolerance test.)

Causes of ST segment depression	
Source	Pathology
cardiac	ischaemia, AS, LVH, intraventricular conduction defect (e.g. LBBB)
non-cardiac	hypokalaemia, digoxin, hypertension

Fig. 12.10 Causes of ST segment depression. (AS, aortic stenosis; LBBB, left bundle branch block; LVH, left ventricular hypertrophy.)

- ST segment depression of more than 1 mm—this should occur in more than one lead and the ST segments should preferably not be upsloping (Fig. 12.9).
- ST segment elevation.
- Chest pain—provided that the pain has the characteristics of angina pain.
- Ventricular arrhythmias.
- Abnormal blood pressure response.

Causes of ST segment depression are listed in Fig. 12.10.

Contraindications to exercise testing

This list includes conditions in which additional stress on the heart may be very hazardous:

- Marked aortic stenosis—gradient greater than 50 mmHg with normal left ventricular function.
- Acute pyrexial or flu-like illness.
- Cardiac failure.
- Unstable angina.
- Second or third degree atrioventricular block.
- Patients unable to walk effectively (e.g. due to severe arthritis or peripheral vascular disease).

Despite adhering to these rules exercise testing does have a mortality rate of approximately 0.5–1/10 000.

In all cases there should be a defibrillator at hand and all the necessary equipment for advanced cardiopulmonary resuscitation.

ECHOCARDIOGRAPHY

Echocardiography is the use of ultrasound to investigate the structure and function of the heart.

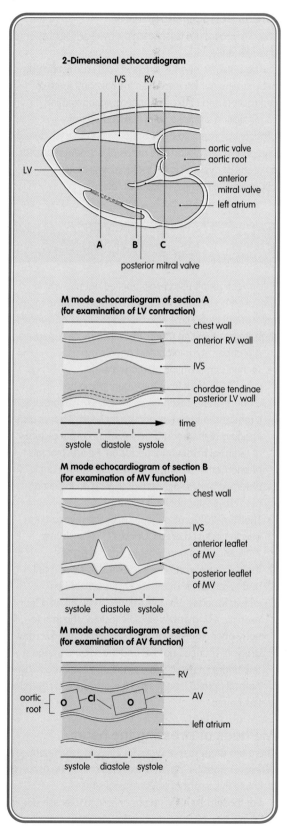

Fig. 12.11 Two-dimensional and M mode echocardiography. The top illustration shows a long axis view of the heart taken from the left parasternal position with the transducer placed at the left lower sternal edge. The B view shows the opening and closing of the mitral valve (MV). The normal valve gives an M shape when opening and closing with time. Left and right ventricular diameters are also measured with this view. The C view shows the aortic valve (AV) leaflets, which make a box shape when opening and closing with time. Left atrial and aortic root measurements can be made here. (Cl, closed; IVS, interventricular septum; LV, left ventricle; O, open; RV, right ventricle.)

The frequency of the waves used is between 1 and 10 MHz (1 MHz = 1 000 000 Hz). The upper limit of audible sound is 20 kHz (1 kHz = 1000 Hz).

The ultrasound waves are generated by a piezoelectric element within the transducer.

The ultrasound waves travel through certain structures (e.g. blood) and are reflected off others (e.g. muscle and bone). The reflected waves are picked up by the transducer and by knowing the time taken for the sound to return and the speed of the waves through the medium, the distance of the reflecting object from the transducer can be calculated.

By rapidly generating waves and detecting reflected waves a picture of the heart can be built up.

M mode echocardiography

The transducer is stationary and records only a single cut through the heart producing an image on a moving page. The result is the activity along that line seen changing with time. This mode of echocardiography is useful for:
- Visualizing the movement of the mitral and aortic valve leaflets.
- Assessing left ventricular dimensions and function.
- Assessing aortic root size.
- Assessing left atrial size.

Two-dimensional echocardiography

The ultrasound generator moves from side to side so a sector of the heart is visualized.

In the echocardiographic examination standard views of the heart are taken (Fig. 12.11) to provide information on:
- Valve structure and function.
- Left ventricular contractility.
- Size of the chambers.
- Congenital cardiac malformations.
- Pericardial disease.

The inadequacies of this approach are:
- The presence of lung between the heart and chest wall precludes ultrasound travel —'poor windows'.
- The posterior part of the heart is furthest from the transducer and may not be viewed adequately, particularly when searching for thrombi and vegetations.

Doppler echocardiography

This uses the principle of the Doppler effect to record blood flow within the heart and great vessels. Doppler effect is the phenomenon where the frequency of ultrasound reflected off moving objects (e.g. blood cells) varies according to the speed and direction of movement. Colour Doppler echocardiography uses different colours depending upon the direction of blood flow, so enabling the operator to assess both the speed and the direction of blood flow.

Doppler echocardiography is used for:
- Assessment of valve stenosis and regurgitation.
- Assessment of atrial and ventricular septal defects, patent ductus arteriosus, and other congenital anomalies.
- Assessment of pulmonary hypertension.

Transoesophageal echocardiography

Transoesophageal echocardiography (TOE) uses a flexible endoscope with a two-dimensional transducer incorporated into the tip. Images are obtained by introducing the transducer into the distal oesophagus. The advantage of TOE is that images are much clearer because the transducer is in close apposition to the heart. Because of this TOE is the investigation of choice for:
- Assessment of intracardiac thrombus—transthoracic echocardiography (TTE) is unreliable.
- Assessment of prosthetic valve function—the planes used in TTE result in a great deal of artefact generated by the prosthesis.
- Assessment of valve vegetations.
- Assessment of congenital heart lesions (e.g. atrial and ventricular septal defects).
- Imaging can be performed in multiple planes whereas TTE is restricted to a few planes.
- TOE can be used intraoperatively during cardiac surgery to provide information on valve function and left ventricular function.

Stress echocardiography

When myocardium is ischaemic it contracts less strongly and efficiently.

The patient's heart is stressed with a drug such as dobutamine, which increases the rate and force of contraction and causes peripheral vasodilatation, so mimicking exercise. With a skilled operator echocardiography images are obtained before, during, and after dobutamine and areas of ischaemia are seen as areas of dyskinesia (or regional wall motion abnormalities), which recover at rest.

MYOCARDIAL PERFUSION IMAGING

This investigation uses radiolabelled agents, which are taken up by the myocardium proportional to local myocardial blood flow. It is more sensitive and specific than exercise testing alone, but much more expensive.

A number of radiolabelled agents are used.
- Technetium-99m labelled agents— (e.g. ^{99m}T-sestamibi). This agent has a half-life of 6 hours and is taken up by perfused myocardium. It remains in the myocardium for several hours and imaging of the heart provides an accurate picture of regional myocardial perfusion. Because of this phenomenon resting and exercise images are obtained on two different days with an injection of ^{99m}Tc-sestamibi for each day.
- Thallium-201 is also taken up by the myocardium only in perfused areas. Unlike ^{99m}Tc-sestamibi, thallium is continually being passed across the cell membrane (i.e. it is extruded by one cell and taken up by another). This redistribution allows for early and late images to be taken after exercise using only a single injection. The image early after exercise (or drug stimulation) shows any areas of reduced uptake and the second image a few hours later will show whether these areas have normal uptake, suggesting the presence of reversible ischaemia

Methods of stressing the heart

There are a number of ways for stressing the heart. Wherever possible physical exercise should be used because this is actual physiological stress.

For those patients who are unable to exercise due to poor mobility, peripheral vascular disease, or respiratory disease pharmacological stress may be used. (Patients who have aortic stenosis or cardiac failure should not have any sort of stress testing.)

The following are commonly used agents pharmacological stress:

- Dipyridamole—this blocks the reabsorption of adenosine into the cells, so increasing intravascular adenosine concentrations. Adenosine is a powerful vasodilator and vasodilates normal coronary arteries, but not diseased coronary arteries. It therefore redistributes blood flow away from diseased vessels. This relative hypoperfusion of diseased areas is picked up by radionucleotide myocardial imaging.
- Adenosine—a direct infusion of adenosine may be used.
- Dobutamine infusion—this drug mimics exercise by increasing myocardial rate and contractility.

Note that both dipyridimole and adenosine are contraindicated in patients who have bronchospasm.

> **Myocardial perfusion imaging is used in the following situations:**
> ○ **If the exercise ECG is equivocal and confirmation of reversible ischaemia is required before coronary angiography.**
> ○ **If the patient cannot perform an exercise ECG due to poor mobility—in this situation a perfusion scan is performed using drugs to stress the heart.**
>
> **In all other situations an exercise ECG is the first investigation.**

Multigated acquisition scanning

Multigated acquisition (MUGA) scanning is a radionucleotide technique for evaluating cardiac function.

Technetium-99m label is used to label the patient's red blood cells.

The amount of radioactivity detected within the left ventricle is proportional to its volume and its degree of contraction during systole will affect this.

The imaging of the cardiac blood pool is synchronized to the ECG trace and each image is identified by its position within the cardiac cycle.

Hundreds of cycles are recorded and an overall assessment of the left ventricular ejection fraction can be made using the averaged values for end-systolic and end-diastolic volume.

MAGNETIC RESONANCE IMAGING

Magnetic resonance imaging (MRI) will soon be widely used in cardiology. It has a number of advantages:

- It is non-invasive.
- It can be gated by an ECG trace, so producing still images from each stage of the cardiac cycle.

Depending upon which imaging mode is used MRI has a number of uses:

- In ischaemic heart disease myocardial perfusion can be assessed using contrast techniques. The coronary arteries can be directly visualized and this has good correlation with conventional angiography. Also myocardial function before and after pharmacological stress can be assessed.
- In structural heart disease MRI can provide a very wide range of soft tissue contrast and detailed structural information.

POSITRON EMISSION TOMOGRAPHY

Positron emission tomography scanning provides images of the metabolic processes of the myocardium. It is used to assess myocardial viability in patients when conventional techniques (radionucleotide perfusion scanning and coronary angiography) have given equivocal results

CARDIAC CATHETERIZATION

This invasive investigation is used when non-invasive techniques are unable to give adequately detailed information on a cardiac lesion.

Technique

Access to the right side of the heart (right heart catheter) is gained by one of the great veins (e.g. femoral, subclavian, or internal jugular vein).

Access to the left side of the heart is gained by a peripheral artery (e.g. femoral, brachial, or radial artery).

In either case the vessel is punctured using a Seldinger needle (a large hollow needle) and a guide wire is passed through the centre of the needle and into the heart using X-ray guidance. Hollow catheters can then be passed over the wire into the great vessels or the desired chamber where a number of investigations may be carried out:

- The pressure in the chamber or vessel can be recorded.
- Oxygen saturation of the blood at that location can be measured.
- Radiopaque dye can be injected via the catheter to provide information depending upon the location of the catheter—if in the ostia of the coronary arteries the anatomy and patency of the coronary arteries can be assessed (coronary angiography); if in the left ventricle the contractility of the ventricle can be assessed by visualizing the manner in which the dye is expelled from the ventricular cavity; if in the aortic root the size and tortuosity of the aortic root can be seen by the outline of the dye within it.

Left heart catheterization and coronary angiography

Indications

This is indicated for patients who:

- Have a positive exercise test or myocardial perfusion scan.
- Give a good history of and have multiple risk factors for ischaemic heart disease.
- Have had a cardiac arrest.
- Have had a cardiac transplantation—there is a high incidence of atherosclerosis after transplant and yearly angiograms are performed.
- Occupational reasons—for patients who have chest pain even if non-invasive tests are negative (e.g. airline pilots).

Note that the list of indications is much more complicated than this, but you only need to have a general idea of the common indications.

Patient preparation

The following must be completed before the procedure:

- A detailed history to ensure that the indications are appropriate and that the patient has no other serious diseases that may affect the decision to proceed. Any history of allergy to iodine must be noted.
- Examination of the patient to ensure that he or she is well. Peripheral pulses must all be felt for and their absence or presence noted. If the femoral approach is to be used the groin area will need to be shaved just before the procedure.
- The procedure must be carefully explained to the patient.
- The risks must be explained.
- Informed consent is obtained.

Left ventriculogram

This is performed to assess left ventricular function. Dye is injected rapidly to fill the left ventricle and X-ray images are obtained of ventricular contraction.

Coronary angiography

The left and right coronary ostia are located in turn and dye is gently injected into the arteries. Several images are obtained of each artery from different angles so a detailed picture of the anatomy of the arteries can be obtained. Images are recorded using X-ray video recording or cine camera.

Complications of coronary angiography

The average mortality and serious complication rate of coronary angiography is 1/1000 cases. The following complications may occur:

- Haemorrhage from the arterial puncture site—this is more common at the femoral site where percutaneous puncture is used; at the brachial site the artery is dissected out and surgically incised and after the procedure the incision is sutured. Firm pressure should be applied to the site of bleeding and a clotting screen performed; rarely operative repair is necessary.
- Formation of a pseudoaneurysm—this results from weakening of the femoral artery wall and may require surgical repair.
- Infection of the puncture site or rarely septicaemia may occur. Blood cultures and intravenous antibiotics may be required.

- Dye reaction—which may range from mild urticaria and a pyrexia to full-blown anaphylactic shock.
- Thrombosis of the artery used—this results in a cold blue foot or hand and necessitates peripheral angiography and a referral to the vascular surgeons.
- Arrhythmias—these may occur during the angiogram due to coronary arterial spasm or occlusion by the catheter. Any form of arrhythmia may occur (ventricular arrhythmias are more common).
- Pericardial tamponade—this is rare and occurs as a result of coronary artery tear or left ventricular tear. The patient becomes acutely cyanosed and hypotensive. Pericardial aspiration is required urgently.
- Displacement of atherosclerotic fragments, which then emolize more distally, resulting in myocardial infarction, cerebrovascular emboli, ischaemic toes, etc.

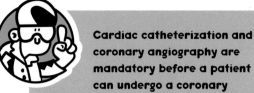

Cardiac catheterization and coronary angiography are mandatory before a patient can undergo a coronary artery bypass operation. It provides detailed information on the severity and location of coronary atherosclerotic lesions without which surgery cannot be undertaken.

Older patients undergoing valve replacement surgery also have coronary angiography before surgery to exclude coexistent coronary artery disease. If this is found, coronary artery bypass may be undertaken at the same time as valve replacement.

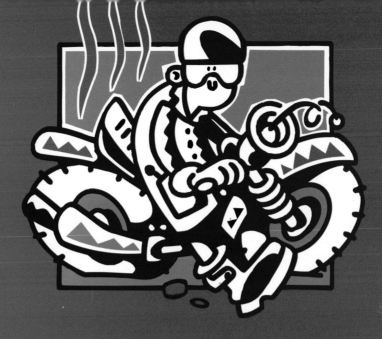

DISEASES AND DISORDERS

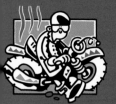

13. Angina Pectoris

DEFINITION OF ANGINA PECTORIS

Angina pectoris is characterized by coronary arterial insufficiency leading to intermittent myocardial ischaemia. (Ischaemia refers to the effect of reduced delivery of oxygen and nutrients to an organ or cell.)

PATHOPHYSIOLOGY OF ANGINA PECTORIS

Myocardial ischaemia occurs when oxygen demand exceeds supply (Fig. 13.1).

Supply may be reduced for a number of reasons:
- Stenotic atheromatous disease of epicardial coronary arteries—the most common cause of angina.
- Thrombosis within the arteries.
- Spasm of normal coronary arteries.
- Inflammation—arteritis.

Demand may be increased for a number of reasons:
- In conditions requiring increased cardiac output —exercise, stress, thyrotoxicosis.
- In conditions necessitating greater cardiac work to maintain an adequate output—aortic stenosis.
- In conditions where peripheral vascular resistance is increased—hypertension.

The rest of this chapter discusses angina due to atherosclerotic narrowing of the coronary arteries because this is the most common cause of angina.

RISK FACTORS FOR CORONARY ARTERY DISEASE

Any modifiable risk factors should be sought and treated to reduce the risk of disease progression and eventual myocardial infarction (Fig. 13.2).

CLINICAL FEATURES OF ANGINA PECTORIS

Symptoms
These include:
- Chest pain—classically a tight, crushing, bandlike pain across the centre of the chest. The pain may radiate to the left arm, throat, or jaw. Precipitating

Factors involved in the development of ischaemia	
Supply factor	**Comments**
coronary blood flow	decreased by fixed stenosis (e.g. atheroma, thrombus); vascular tone—depends upon a number of factors including endothelium-dependent relaxing factor (nitric oxide), prostaglandins, and autonomic nervous system input
oxygen carrying capacity	reduced in anaemia and carboxyhaemaglobinaemia
Demand factor	**Comments**
heart rate	increased by exercise, emotion, tachyarrhythmias, outflow obstruction, hypertension, etc
contractility	decreased by rest and negatively inotropic and chronotropic agents (e.g. β-blockers); increased by exertion and positive inotropes (e.g. adrenaline)
wall tension	increased by left ventricular dilation (e.g. nocturnal angina)

Fig. 13.1 Factors involved in the development of ischaemia.

Risk factors for coronary artery disease
Non-modifiable risk factors
age—risk increases with age; older patients have a higher risk and therefore a potentially greater risk reduction if modifiable risk factors are treated sex—men > women (incidence in women increases rapidly after menopause) family history—this is a strong risk factor even when known genetic diseases (e.g. familial hypercholesterolaemia) are excluded
Modifiable risk factors
hypertension diabetes mellitus smoking hypercholesterolaemia—important studies include MRFIT, Helsinki Heart Study (*N Engl J Med* 317), SSSS (*Lancet* 344), WOSCOPS (*N Engl J Med* 333), CARE (*N Engl J Med* 335) and LIPID (*N Engl J Med* 339)
Other risk factors currently being researched
fibrinogen homocysteine low levels of antioxidants insulin resistance short of overt diabetes mellitus

Fig. 13.2 Risk factors for coronary artery disease. (CARE, Cholesterol and Recurrent Events Trial; LIPID, Long-term Intervention with Pravastatin in Ischaemic Heart Disease; SSSS, Scandinavian Simvastatin Survival Study; WOSCOPS, West of Scotland Coronary Prevention Study.)

factors include exercise, anxiety, and cold air. As the coronary artery narrowing worsens the amount of stress required to produce angina reduces and the pain may occur even at rest or on minimal exertion. Relieving factors include rest and nitrates.

- Dyspnoea—often experienced. This occurs when the ischaemic myocardium becomes dysfunctional with an increase in left ventricular filling pressure and, if severe, progression to pulmonary oedema.
- Fatigue—may be a manifestation of angina, which should be suspected if it occurs abnormally early into exercise and resolves rapidly at rest or to nitrates.

Most patients will have no obvious signs on examination. The patient may be breathless or sweaty. There may be a tachycardia due to anxiety.

There may also be evidence of an underlying cause:
- Hypertension
- Corneal arcus or xanthelasma—suggesting hypercholesterolaemia.
- Nicotine staining of the fingers.
- Aortic stenosis.
- Abnormal tachyarrhythmia.
- Anaemia.

There may be evidence of cardiac failure (third heart sound, bilateral basal crepitations, and possibly peripheral oedema due to fluid retention).

Important points when diagnosing angina are:
- A sudden increase in exertional angina may be due to rupture of an atheromatous plaque in the coronary artery, which causes a step decrease in its luminal diameter; the condition may progress to full infarction.
- Oesophageal pain is also relieved by nitrates.
- Chest pain on exertion can also be musculoskeletal in origin—obtain objective evidence of myocardial ischaemia before giving an opinion.
- Any form of chest discomfort, even if atypical, could be angina, especially if it is related to effort.

INVESTIGATION OF ANGINA PECTORIS

Resting electrocardiography
A normal resting ECG may occur even in individuals who have very severe angina.

Signs of angina on the resting ECG include:
- T wave flattening.
- T wave inversion.
- ST segment depression.
- Partial or complete left bundle branch block.

Stress testing

There are many methods of stress testing. All aim to place the myocardium under stress and increase oxygen demand and therefore precipitate ischaemia, which can be detected in a number of ways.

Remember that precipitation of ischaemia is potentially hazardous and therefore all these tests should be performed with facilities for resuscitation close at hand.

Exercise electrocardiography

The patient is made to walk on a treadmill that becomes incrementally faster and steeper at fixed time intervals. ECG monitoring is used throughout the test and the presence of horizontal ST depression of greater the 1 mm suggests the presence of angina. (If the ST depression is >2 mm strongly suggests angina.) Exercise ECGs are only 70% specific and 70% sensitive and are less reliable in women than men.

Stress myocardial perfusion imaging

The exercise test is performed as above, but a radionucleotide is injected at peak exercise and the patient is encouraged to continue exercising for at least another 30 s. This allows perfused myocardium to pick up the radionucleotide (any ischaemic myocardium will not pick it up due to poor perfusion). Images of tracer uptake are performed at this stage and also after rest some time later (when the ischaemia has resolved and the affected myocardium has had a chance to take up the tracer). Comparison of the two images provides information on the site of reversible ischaemia.

Pharmacological nuclear stress testing

This is used for patients who are unable to exercise adequately due to peripheral vascular disease, arthritis, or chronic obstructive airways disease or asthma.

Agents used include dobutamine, dipyridimole, adenosine, and a new agent arbutamine (which simulates physical exercise more closely and is given as an infusion) the rate of which is determined by the patient's own haemodynamic response to the drug.

Stress echocardiography

Imaging of the cardiac muscle at rest and immediately after exercise or dobutamine allows accurate definition of areas of dysfunction secondary to ischaemia. In addition any valve disorders and left ventricular hypertrophy can be diagnosed.

Coronary angiography

This is used in patients who have positive stress tests and in patients who have negative stress tests in whom the diagnosis of angina is still suspected as stress tests may give false-negative results.

Coronary angiography is the most specific and sensitive test of coronary artery anatomical lesions.

An arterial puncture is made under local anaesthetic in the femoral, brachial, or radial artery, and a guide wire is passed under X-ray control to the aortic root. A series of catheters is used to locate the right and left coronary ostia and radio-opaque dye is injected into each in turn. Images are taken from several angles to obtain a full view of all branches of the two coronary arteries.

Information on left ventricular function is obtained by injection of dye into the left ventricle rapidly to fill it. The rate at which the dye is expelled and the pattern of left ventricular contraction can be seen and gives an assessment of function.

Rapid pacing during cardiac catheterization may provoke ischaemia as judged by:
- ST depression.
- Increase in left ventricular end-diastolic pressure.
- Lactate evolution into the coronary sinus.

Syndrome X

This is the term given to a group of patients (mostly middle-aged women) who have the following characteristics:
- Symptoms of angina pectoris.
- Positive exercise ECG.
- Normal coronary arteries at coronary angiography.

Possible causes for this are:
- Coronary artery spasm.
- Microvascular abnormalities.

The treatment for this syndrome is nitrates and calcium channel antagonists, and the prognosis is good.

MANAGEMENT OF ANGINA PECTORIS

Management of angina involves two areas that are addressed simultaneously:
- Management of any modifiable risk factors.
- Management of the angina itself.

Management of the risk factors

Ban smoking. Patients who smoke should at all stages be actively discouraged to smoke. All health professionals should be involved and positive encouragement, advice on the complications of smoking, and information about self-help groups should all be made available to smokers.

Hypertension should be diagnosed and aggressively treated until the blood pressure is below 140/80 mmHg if possible. Many hypertensive patients are undertreated and regular follow-up is required to ensure this does not happen.

Diabetes mellitus should be tightly controlled and often endocrinology follow-up is needed to ensure that control is well maintained.

Hypercholesterolaemia should also be treated (Fig. 13.3). Some centres recommend that patients who have coronary artery disease should have total cholesterol maintained under 5 mmol/L with low-density lipoprotein maintained below 3 mmol/L. Others may have slightly higher or lower recommended levels. Diet therapy should be tried first, but it is vital that after a fixed period of dietary modification (e.g. 3 months) the fasting lipid profile is checked again and pharmacological agents used if the target levels have not been attained. The trials mentioned in Fig. 13.2 should be read because they have dramatically altered the way hypercholesterolaemia is treated.

Treatment of the angina
Drug therapy

The main drugs used in the treatment of angina are aspirin, β-blockers (β-adrenoceptor antagonist), calcium channel antagonists, nitrates, and potassium channel openers.

Aspirin

Aspirin acts to reduce platelet aggregation, which is a risk factor for the development and progression of atherosclerotic plaques.

β-Blockers

These agents are negatively inotropic and chronotropic and therefore reduce myocardial oxygen demand swinging the balance of demand and supply. They are also effective antihypertensive agents and in some patients can perform a dual role reducing the need for multiple drug therapy. Remember that β-blockers are contraindicated in:
- Unstable cardiac failure.
- Asthma.
- Peripheral vascular disease—a relative contraindication and the more β_1-selective agents may be used (e.g. bisoprolol).

Other side effects include:
- Nightmares—use a non-fat soluble agent (e.g. atenolol).
- Loss of sympathetic response to hypoglycaemia —use a more cardioselective agent.
- Postural hypotension—especially in elderly patients who should start on a small dose initially.

Calcium channel antagonists

The slowing of calcium influx to the myocardial cells results in a negative inotropic response. The blockade of calcium channels in peripheral arteries results in relaxation and therefore vasodilatation This improves blood flow. The blockade of calcium channels in the atrioventricular node increases the refractory period and therefore slows the heart rate. Agents in this group have actions on one or more of these areas and this affects the way they should be used:
- Nifedipine dilates both coronary and peripheral vessels and can be used as an antihypertensive and antianginal drug. Main side effects are flushing, reflex tachycardia, and ankle oedema.
- Diltiazem dilates coronary arteries and has some negative inotropic and chronotropic effects. It is therefore a good antianginal drug. It has less effect on peripheral vessels. It causes less flushing and oedema and no reflex tachycardia.
- Verapamil has almost no peripheral effects; its main effects are on the atrioventricular node and myocardium, therefore can be used as an antianginal agent, but is used mainly as an antiarrhythmic.

Drugs used to treat hypercholesterolaemia

Drug	Notes	Examples	Action	Indication	Adverse effects	Information from clinical trials
HMG CoA reductase inhibitors	mainstay of treatment; generally well tolerated and effective; taken only once daily	simvastatin, pravastatin, atorvastatin, cerivastatin	inhibition of HMG CoA reductase, the rate-limiting intrahepatic enzyme in cholesterol synthesis; intracellular cholesterol levels fall leading to upregulation of apolipoprotein B and E receptors on the cell surface, resulting in increased clearance of these from the blood; LDL cholesterol levels fall	most effective cholesterol lowering agents available and so first-line therapy	hepatotoxicity (LFTs should be checked before therapy and then 6-monthly); myositis —patients may complain of muscle tenderness (creatine kinase should be checked and if significantly elevated the agent should be discontinued)	many studies show that statins reduce cardiovascular mortality of patients who have and do not have a previous history of coronary artery disease (e.g. SSSS study, CARE study, WOSCOPS and LIPID study)
fibric acid derivatives	also reduce fibrinogen	clofibrate, gemfibrozil, fenofibrate	increased lipoprotein lipase activity leading to decreased VLDL; there is a significant reduction in the blood triglyceride levels and a less significant decrease in blood cholesterol concentration; there is also reduced platelet aggregation	if statins not tolerated or contraindicated or severe hypertriglyceridaemia	non-specific gastrointestinal symptoms; occasional myositis, especially if combined with a statin	Helsinki Heart Study showed that when compared with placebo gemfibrozil reduced cardiovascular mortality in hypercholesterolaemic men at 5-year follow-up
bile acid sequestrants		cholestyramine	interrupt enterohepatic recycling of bile acids by binding them in the gut from where they are excreted in the faeces; bile acid synthesis increases resulting in decreased intracellular cholesterol and therefore upregulation of apolipoprotein B and E receptors	some familial hyperlipidaemias	gastrointestinal (e.g. reflux, nausea)	reduces lipids, but no mortality rate data
nicotinic acid	rarely tolerated		decreases hepatic synthesis of VLDL	some familial hyperlipidaemias	flushing, dizziness, headache, palpitations, pruritus, nausea, vomiting, impaired liver function, rashes	flushing, hepatic toxicity
probucol	not available		possible antioxidant effect on LDL with mild cholesterol reduction			gastrointestinal, long QT interval
vitamin E	normal vitamin		antioxidant action counteracts LDL effects in arterial wall		none in μg or mg doses	ongoing
fish oil	normal component of diet	Maxepa	populations on traditional high fish oil diets have low incidence of coronary disease		nausea, belching	ongoing
folic acid	normal vitamin		decreases homocysteine		none	ongoing

Fig. 13.3 Drugs used to treat hypercholesterolaemia. (CAD, coronary artery disease; HMG CoA, 3-hydroxy-3-methylglutaryl coenzyme A; LDL, low density lipoprotein; LFTs, liver function tests; VLDL, very low density lipoprotein; SSSS, Scandinavian Simvastatin Survival Study.)

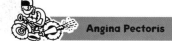

- Amlodipine is a long-acting agent with actions similar to those of nifedipine. It is an effective antianginal and antihypertensive agent.

Nitrates

These act by conversion to nitric oxide, which is a potent vasodilator (so mimicking the endothelial release of nitric oxide). The vasodilatation affects:

- Veins—shifting blood from the central compartment (heart, pulmonary vessels) to peripheral veins.
- Arteries—reducing arterial pressure.
- Coronary arteries—improving myocardial perfusion.

There are a variety of preparations:

- Sublingual—glyceryl trinitrate or isosorbide dinitrate can both be taken sublingually from where they are absorbed and rapidly enter the blood. There is no risk of tolerance. Glyceryl trinitrate tablets should be changed every 6 months because they have a short shelf life. Sublingual sprays do not have this problem.
- Transdermal—these take the form of patches or cream that allow the drug to be absorbed through the skin. Care should be taken to vary the location of the application each day.
- Oral nitrates—these may be once, twice, or three times a day dosages.

All nitrates cause headache and flushing because of their vasodilatory action.
Tolerance may develop to the oral and transdermal preparations; therefore a nitrate-free period of 6 hours should be arranged by removing patches overnight or taking the twice daily preparations at 8 a.m. and 2 p.m.

Potassium channel openers

There are many families of potassium channels found in cardiac and vascular smooth muscle and these are still incompletely understood. Nicorandil is a potassium channel opener that has been increasingly used to treat angina. The action of potassium channel openers results in venous and arterial dilatation (coronary and systemic). Potassium channel openers also act to precondition the myocardium against ischaemia, so limiting the area of myocardium vulnerable to ischaemia.

Side effects of potassium channel openers are similar to those of nitrates (i.e. headache and flushing). Tolerance is not a problem.

Management plan for angina pectoris

A possible plan of action is therefore:

- Prescribe all patients aspirin
- Prescribe a β-blocker if not contraindicated.
- If β-blockade fails to control the symptoms or is contraindicated there is a choice to either start a calcium antagonist and be prepared to add a long-acting nitrate or nicorandil if the effect is still insufficient, or prescribe nicorandil, which has effects similar to those produced by a combination of calcium antagonist and nitrate.

When diagnosing ischaemia, remember that:
- Angina patients have additional ischaemic episodes that do not cause pain —called 'silent ischaemia' and detectable on Holter monitoring.
- Silent ischaemia is more common in diabetics who have autonomic neuropathy.
- Drug therapy needs to be tailored to the characteristics of the individual patient.

Revascularization

There are two main ways of improving myocardial blood supply and coronary angiography is required to make the judgement:

- Percutaneous transluminal angioplasty (PTCA) forces the lumen open by means of an inflated intraluminal balloon; this can be reinforced by stenting.
- Coronary artery bypass surgery (CABG).

Percutaneous transluminal coronary angioplasty

Percutaneous transluminal coronary angioplasty (PTCA) achieves revascularization by the inflation of a small balloon placed across a stenotic lesion. The procedure is carried out in the catheter laboratory under local anaesthetic.

A guide-wire is passed into the aorta via the femoral or brachial artery and the balloon catheter is passed over it. Once the balloon catheter has been positioned across the stenotic plaque to be treated the balloon is inflated.

Advantages of PTCA

The advantages of this technique over coronary artery bypass grafting (CABG) are as follows:

- No general anaesthetic is needed.
- The patient does not need a cardiopulmonary bypass.
- Patients unfit for CABG can still be treated.
- Patients who have clotting disorders or who have recently had thrombolysis can be treated in an emergency.
- If PTCA is unsuccessful CABG can still be performed (whereas a second CABG operation carries a much higher risk).

Disadvantages of PTCA

Patients who have left main stem disease are unsuitable, as are patients who have multivessel disease and tortuous vessels. Patient selection is therefore important.

The restenosis rate is much higher than with CABG—approximately 30% within the first 6 months after PTCA.

Complications of PTCA

These include:

- Myocardial infarction—secondary to thrombosis, spasm of the coronary artery, or dissection of the coronary artery by the balloon.
- Coronary artery perforation.
- Arrhythmias.
- Dye reactions
- Haemorrhage or infection at the puncture site.

PTCA with coronary artery stenting

In the past 10 years the use of stents in conjunction with PTCA has dramatically increased. These have been shown to reduce the risk of restenosis after PTCA.

Stents are flexible metal cylindrical structures, usually with a mesh or coil design. They are initially loaded in a compressed form over the deflated balloon and expand when the balloon is inflated at the site of stenosis.

Thrombosis at the site of stenting may occur and is partly prevented by the use of intravenous heparin and antiplatelet aggregation agents (Fig. 13.4).

Antiplatelet agents used to prevent thrombosis following PTCA +/– stenting		
Class of drug and examples	**Action**	**Side effects**
NSAIDs (e.g. aspirin)	irreversible inactivation of cyclooxygenase—within platelets this enzyme is needed for the production of thromboxane (a stimulator of platelet aggregation)	gastritis (possibly with ulcer formation and bleeding), renal impairment, bronchospasm, rashes
platelet ADP receptor antagonists (e.g. ticlopidine, clopidogrel)	when activated the adenyl cyclase-coupled ADP receptor causes binding of fibrinogen to the platelet and initiation of thrombus formation —this is irreversibly inhibited by these agents	haemorrhage, diarrhoea, nausea, neutropenia (more so with ticlodipine), hepatic dysfunction
platelet membrane glycoprotein IIb/IIIa receptors (abciximab is a monoclonal antibody that binds to and blocks this receptor)	the Gp IIa/IIIb platelet receptor binds fibrinogen, von Willebrand's factor, and other adhesive molecules—blockade therefore inhibits platelet aggregation and thrombus formation	haemorrhage

Fig. 13.4 Antiplatelet agents used to prevent thrombosis following PTCA +/– stenting. (ADP, adenosine diphosphate; NSAIDs, non-steroidal anti-inflammatory drugs.)

Coronary artery bypass grafting

Coronary artery bypass grafting aims to achieve revascularization by bypassing a stenotic lesion using grafts.

The patient undergoes a full general anaesthetic and the heart is exposed using a median sternotomy incision and sternal retractors.

Cardiopulmonary bypass is achieved by inserting a cannula into the right atrium and another into the proximal aorta. The two cannulas are connected to the bypass machine, which oxygenates the venous blood from the right atrium and feeds it back to the aorta.

The heart is stopped using cooling and cardioplegic solutions.

Vein grafts harvested from the great saphenous vein or arterial grafts are used to bypass the occlusive coronary lesions.

A number of arteries may be used for grafting including:
- Left and right internal mammary arteries.
- Radial arteries.
- Gastroepiploic artery.
- Inferior epigastric artery.

The last two in this list are used much less often than the first two.

Arterial grafts have the advantage of having much lower rates of reocclusion.

Complications of CABG

These are:
- Death—mortality rates are approximately 1% in good centres.
- Myocardial infarction, stroke, peripheral thromboembolism.
- Wound infection.
- Complications related to cardiopulmonary bypass —these are related to the haemodilution involved and the exposure of the blood to manmade materials in the oxygenating process, and include clotting and pulmonary abnormalities, and impaired cognitive function.

Minimally invasive coronary artery bypass grafting

Minimally invasive CABG (MICABG) is a new technique that involves a smaller incision, usually a left anterior mini-thoracotomy. The left or right internal mammary artery is used to graft the occluded vessel (usually the left anterior descending coronary artery because this is situated within easy reach).

Cardiopulmonary bypass is not used—instead the heart is slowed using β-blockers and a specifically designed instrument is used to immobilize the small area around the anastomosis.

Benefits of MICABG

Compared with traditional CABG, MICABG has the benefits of:
- A rapid recovery because of smaller scar.
- No need for cardiopulmonary bypass.

Disadvantages of MICABG

Compared with traditional CABG, MICABG has the following disadvantages:
- It sometimes takes longer to carry out.
- Multiple stenoses cannot be bypassed so it is currently only suitable for patients who require only one or two grafts.
- Lesions of the right coronary or circumflx arteries are more difficult to graft.

UNSTABLE ANGINA

This condition is one of the acute coronary syndromes.

The pathophysiology underlying unstable angina involves rupture of an atherosclerotic plaque within the coronary artery and the subsequent formation of a thrombus over this. The result is a rapid reduction in the size of the lumen of the vessel.

A marked change in symptoms occurs. The patient who has angina on exertion only suddenly develops an increase in severity of the pain and eventually pain at rest.

Management

The following management plan should be followed:
- Admit the patient to the coronary care unit for observation and strict bed rest—remember that if the thrombus extends and completely occludes the vessel lumen a myocardial infarction will occur.
- Provide analgesia with intravenous diamorphine (2.5–5 mg intravenously) if required to calm the patient and relieve pain—remember to give metoclopramide too.

- Give aspirin—it has been shown to reduce the incidence of myocardial infarction and death in patients who have unstable angina (300 mg soluble aspirin).
- Give an intravenous infusion of nitrates (e.g. glyceryl trinitrate 0.5–2 mg/hour)—to dilate the coronary arteries and reduce the load on the heart by peripheral vasodilatation and venodilatation. The blood pressure will drop so it should be carefully monitored.
- Give intravenous heparin as a 24-hour infusion (or subcutaneous low-molecular-weight heparin) to prevent further thrombus formation. Intravenous heparin has the disadvantage that the activated partial thromboplastin time needs to be monitored to ensure that it does not become too high and lead to haemorrhage. Low-molecular-weight heparins are given at doses according to patient weight and no such measurements are required. There is evidence to suggest that the low-molecular-weight heparins are more effective than intravenous heparin.
- Once the patient is more stable start oral antianginal therapy and arrange early angiography if appropriate.

Low molecular weight heparins

The main events leading to unstable angina and MI are the rupture of the atherosclerotic plaque and then subsequent thrombus formation over the plaque. Thrombus formation requires both platelet activation and aggregation and fibrin deposition and thrombin generation.

Heparin comprises a highly heterogeneous group of compounds—all are proteoglycans, but they differ in their constituent sugar units and in their molecular weight.

Heparin acts to alter antithrombin, which becomes much more effective in inhibiting thrombin and the coagulation factors Xa and IXa.

The problems with heparin administration for unstable angina are as follows:
- To maintain a constant effect heparin must be given as an intravenous infusion. Therefore the patient must be an inpatient and be relatively immobile.
- During this time the activated partial thromboplastin time must be regularly monitored to ensure that the effect of heparin is not too little (rendering the drug ineffective) or too great (leading to a risk of haemorrhage).

Side effects of heparin include osteoporosis and thrombocytopenia.

Low molecular weight heparins form a more uniform group of heparins with 13–22 sugar residues. They have high bioavailibility after subcutaneous injection and a longer half-life. They also have a more predictable anticoagulant effect than conventional heparin.

The benefits of low molecular weight heparin are:
- They can be given as twice daily subcutaneous injections instead of as a continuous infusion.
- The dose is adjusted according to patient weight and the anticoagulant effect is sufficiently predictable that regular monitoring is not required.
- There is a lower risk of osteoporosis and thrombocytopenia.

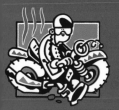

14. Acute Myocardial Infarction

DEFINITION OF ACUTE MYOCARDIAL INFARCTION

Acute myocardial infarction (MI) is the term used for cell death secondary to ischaemia. The most common cause of MI is atherosclerotic narrowing of the coronary arteries. The immediate precursor to MI is rupture of an atherosclerotic plaque and the formation of thrombus over the plaque resulting in rapid occlusion of the vessel.

Depending upon the rate of vessel occlusion (if an atherosclerotic plaque grows slowly over months collateral vessels develop and protect the myocardium) and the degree of occlusion of the vessel by thrombus a number of clinical conditions can result from plaque rupture. These conditions are termed the acute coronary syndromes.

Acute MI is the most serious of this spectrum of acute illnesses (Fig. 14.1).

For simplicity, and to make the management algorithm work (see below), these are divided into two categories:

- ST elevation.
- No ST elevation.

All these syndromes present as severe central chest pain of typical cardiac type (see Chapter 1), and patients usually present at the accident and emergency department with one of the following:

- Severe angina—there is a history of angina and the pain usually subsides spontaneously with rest and nitrates without permanent change to the ECG or evidence of activation of coagulation or myocardial damage.
- A sudden increase in exertional angina—there is rupture of an atheromatous plaque in the coronary artery, which causes a step decrease in its luminal diameter; the pain usually subsides spontaneously with rest and nitrates, without permanent change to the ECG or evidence of activation of coagulation or myocardial damage. The condition may progress to full infarction.
- Widespread subendocardial ischaemia—ST depression may be present in all ECG leads except AVR. This is a manifestation of critical stenoses in all three coronary arteries. There is no evidence of activation of coagulation, or myocardial damage, but the prognosis is very poor without emergency coronary artery bypass grafting (CABG).
- Unstable angina due to coronary arterial thrombosis—there is no ST elevation, but microinfarcts may be occurring due to embolization of thrombi from the site of plaque rupture downstream.
- Non-Q wave infarction—this is necrosis caused by thrombotic coronary artery occlusion in which the myocardial cell death is confined to the endocardial layers and is not full thickness. It occurs either because the occluded artery is a relatively small branch, or because there is good collateral flow around the occluded vessel, or because thrombolysis for ST elevation has been early and effective.
- Q wave infarction—this follows necrosis through the whole thickness of the ventricular wall, leaving permanent Q waves on the ECG (Fig. 14.2).

Acute coronary syndromes in descending order of severity
Q wave infarction
non-Q wave infarction
unstable angina due to coronary arterial thrombosis
widespread subendocardial ischaemia
sudden increase in severity of exertional angina
severe angina episode in a patient who has exertional angina

Fig. 14.1 Acute coronary syndromes in order of severity (indicated by arrow).

CLINICAL FEATURES OF ACUTE MYOCARDIAL INFARCTION

History

The history is very important because it provides clues about the severity of the infarction and the time of onset (important when deciding on therapy). The following are classical features of the history of acute MI.

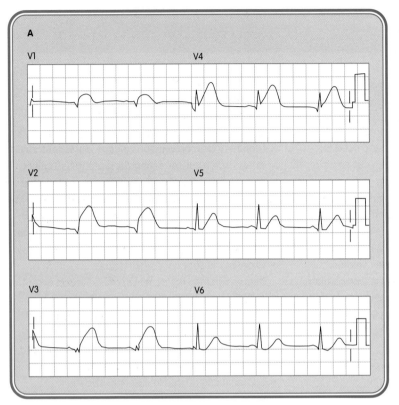

A

V1   V4

V2   V5

V3   V6

Fig. 14.2 (A) ECG showing acute anterior MI. **(B)** ECG 24 hours after anterior MI. Note the resolution of the ST elevation and the development of Q waves. The loss of the R wave in this ECG suggests that a significant left ventricle muscle mass has undergone necrosis.

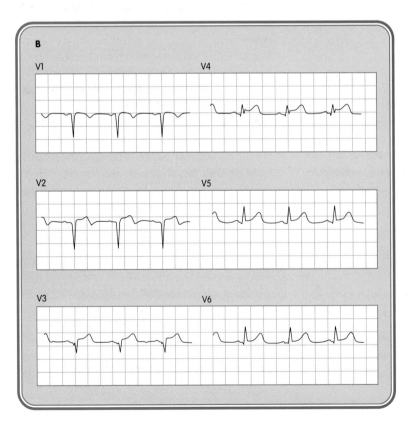

B

V1   V4

V2   V5

V3   V6

Presenting complaint

The main presenting complaint is of chest pain. The following characteristics are common:

- Usually severe in nature.
- Normally lasts at least 30 min.
- Usually tight, crushing, and bandlike in nature.
- Retrosternal in location.
- May radiate to the left arm, throat, or jaw.
- Associated features include sweating, breathlessness, and nausea.
- Elderly patients may have relatively little pain, but may present with features of left ventricular failure (profound breathlessness) or syncope.

Past medical history

Important features include a history of angina or intermittent chest pain that often increases in severity or frequency in the few weeks preceding this event.

Risk factors for ischaemic heart disease are smoking, hypertension, diabetes mellitus, hypercholesterolaemia, positive family history. (Although some of these do not belong in this section of the clerking it is important not to forget these and therefore easier to ask about them all together at the same time).

The patient may have a history of previous MIs or of cardiac intervention such as angiography, percutaneous transluminal angioplasty (PTCA), or coronary artery bypass grafts (CABG).

Also ask about any contraindication for thrombolysis at this stage (see p. 104).

Examination

On inspection the patient is often extremely anxious and distressed and will often be restless. He or she may be in severe pain. Breathlessness suggests the presence of pulmonary oedema, as does the presence of pink frothy sputum. The patient may be pale, clammy, and sweaty, suggesting a degree of cardiogenic shock. Look for scars of previous surgery.

Cardiovascular system

The pulse may be tachycardic secondary to anxiety or left ventricular failure or it may be bradycardic in the case of an inferior MI where the right coronary artery is occluded and the atrioventricular node (which is supplied by the right coronary artery in 90% of people) is affected.

The blood pressure may be normal. In some patients it may be high and this may be due to anxiety. If there is cardiogenic shock the blood pressure may be low.

The jugular venous pressure may be elevated in cases of congestive cardiac failure or in pure right ventricular infarction.

Examination of the praecordium may reveal the following:

- A displaced diffuse apex in cases of left ventricular failure.
- In anterior infarction a paradoxical systolic outward movement of the ventricular wall may be felt parasternally.
- Audible murmurs.
- The murmur of mitral regurgitation—may occur as a new murmur due to rupture of the papillary muscle.
- A pericardial rub—may be audible in some patients because it is not uncommon for an MI to be complicated by pericarditis.
- A fourth heart sound (Fig. 14.3)—common in MI due to reduction of left ventricular compliance.
- A third heart sound—occurs in the presence of left ventricular failure.
- Further evidence of cardiac failure (e.g. bilateral basal crepitations, peripheral oedema and poor peripheral perfusion).

Notes on third and fourth heart sounds			
Heart sound	Mechanism	When heard	Causes
fourth	represents atrial contribution to ventricular filling	heard in any condition that causes a 'stiff' left ventricular wall	hypertension, aortic stenosis, acute myocardial infarction
third	rapid filling of the ventricle as soon as the mitral valve opens	normal finding in the young and heard in conditions where there is fluid overload of the ventricle	mitral regurgitation, ventricular septal defect, left ventricular failure, myocardial infarction

Fig. 14.3 Notes on third and fourth heart sounds.

INVESTIGATION OF ACUTE MYOCARDIAL INFARCTION

Blood tests
Indicators of myocardial damage
Creatine kinase
The MB isoenzyme of creatine kinase (CK) increases and falls within 72 hours. (The source of CK-MB isoenzyme is cardiac muscle, whereas CK-MM is found in skeletal muscle and CK-BB is in brain and kidney. Many laboratories only provide total CK measurements for routine use and this is not specific.) The CK-MB isoenzyme does not begin to increase until at least 4 hours after infarction and is therefore not used to make the initial diagnosis in most cases.

Troponin T
This is a relatively new test and is not yet widely available. It is more cardiospecific than the rest and increases rapidly, remaining elevated for 2 weeks. In patients who have unstable angina marginally high levels of troponin T indicate a high likelihood of subsequent infarction.

Aspartate aminotransferase
(serum glutamic oxaloacetic transaminase)
This is less specific. The levels increase and fall within 4–6 days with peak levels at 24 hours. Other causes of elevated aspartate aminotransferase levels are hepatic disorders, thrombotic conditions (e.g. pulmonary embolus) and skeletal muscle injury.

Lactate dehydrogenase
Lactate dehydrogenase is not cardiospecific and has an even more delayed response with a peak at 4 days and remaining elevated for 1–2 weeks.

Hydroxybutyrate dehydrogenase is a more cardiospecific isoform of lactate dehydrogenase and shows the same time scale of response.

Renal function and electrolytes
These are important in all patients who have MI. Renal function may be deranged or may worsen due to poor renal perfusion in cardiogenic shock. Hypokalaemia may predispose to arrhythmias and must be corrected because acute MI is in itself a proarrhythmogenic condition.

Blood glucose
Diabetes mellitus must be aggressively controlled after MI and all patients who have diabetes mellitus benefit from insulin therapy either using an intravenous sliding scale or if stable four times daily subcutaneous insulin.

Full blood count
Anaemia may precipitate an acute MI in a patient who has angina. There is often a leucocytosis after acute MI.

Serum cholesterol
This should be measured within 24–48 hours of an MI —otherwise it may be forgotten. Hypercholesterolaemia is a risk factor for MI and should therefore be treated in all these patients. Cholesterol level falls to an artificially low level 24 hours after MI, so a true reading can then only be obtained 2 months after MI.

Electrocardiography
The ECG is the main diagnostic test in acute MI and it is therefore important to have a thorough knowledge of the ECG appearances of different types of MI. Delay in the diagnosis wastes precious time because thrombolysis should be given as soon as possible for maximum benefit.

Classical ECG changes of a full-thickness MI are as follows:
- ST segment elevation—this is due to full-thickness myocardial injury and may appear within minutes of the onset of infarction; it is almost always present by 24 hours. The criteria for acute thrombolysis are a good history and ST segment elevation greater than 1 mm in two or more consecutive leads. Reciprocal ST segment depression may be present at the same time and represents the mirror image of the ST elevation as seen from the opposite side of the heart.
- Over 24 hours the ST elevation resolves and the T waves begin to invert.
- Q waves develop within 24–72 hours after MI.

Persistent elevation of ST segments after 1 week indicate either reinfarction or a left ventricular aneurysm.

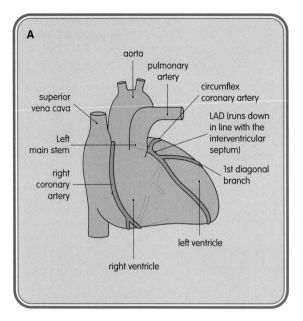

B	Localizing ECG changes	
Location of MI	ECG changes	
anterior (LAD)	ST elevation in leads V1–4	
inferior (RCA or circumflex coronary artery)	ST elevation in leads II, III, AVF	
lateral (circumflex coronary artery)	ST elevation in leads V4–6	
posterior (RCA or circumflex coronary artery)	prominent R wave in V1 and V2 with ST depression (mirror image of anterior MI)	
anterolateral (proximal LAD) above diagonal branch	ST elevation V1–6	
right ventricular infarction (suspect in inferior or posterior MI)	perform right-sided ECG using lead V1 (as normal), leads V3–6 placed on the right side, limb leads as normal	

Fig 14.4 (A) Location of coronary arteries. Note the left anterior descending coronary artery branch (LAD) supplies the anterior aspect of the heart (the left ventricle and the septum), the right coronary artery (RCA) supplies the inferoposterior aspect, and the circumflex supplies the lateral part of the left ventricle. **(B)** Localizing ECG changes.

ECG changes in non-Q wave myocardial infarction

These are variable and the absence of Q waves does not necessarily indicate that full-thickness infarction has not occurred. (The conventional view was that this represented subendocardial damage only.)

The ECG changes tend to be in the form of persistent T wave inversion accompanied by an increase in cardiac enzymes.

Chest radiography

This should be performed on all patients who have acute MI. Points to note are:

- Widening of the mediastinum—suggests a likelihood of aortic dissection, which is an absolute contraindication for thrombolysis.
- Signs of pulmonary oedema—signify the need for antifailure therapy (intravenous diuretics, oxygen, and possibly a nitrate infusion).
- An enlarged heart—suggests cardiac failure.

Echocardiography

This is not a first-line investigation, but is very useful in the first week to assess left ventricular function or investigate valve lesions (mitral regurgitation may occur after MI as a result of papillary muscle infarction).

MANAGEMENT OF ACUTE MYOCARDIAL INFARCTION

Acute MI is a medical emergency and therefore you must know its acute management thoroughly (Fig. 14.5). It is one of the few occasions in an examination when you will be expected to know the doses of drugs given.

The management of MI has changed dramatically over the past 10 years and as a result of these changes the mortality rate after MI has fallen significantly. In addition to knowing the management it is useful (and impressive) if you have a knowledge of the many trials that have provided evidence for these changes and these will be mentioned in this chapter.

Thrombolysis

A number of large prospective double-blind placebo controlled trials have shown that thrombolysis reduces mortality rate after MI, for example the Italian GISSI

Acute management of acute AMI
administer oxygen via a facial mask
give the patient soluble aspirin 300 mg in water
establish IV access and connect patient to cardiac monitor
if patient is distressed or in pain give diamorphine 2.5–5 mg IV with 10 mg metoclopramide
if patient satisfies the criteria for thrombolysis and has no contraindications administer thrombolysis: streptokinase 1.5 million units in 100 ml normal saline IV over 1 hour or rt-PA if the patient has ever had streptokinase before or is young (<65) patient and has an anterior MI
administer intravenous atenolol 5 mg over 10 minutes and if tolerated after 10 minutes repeat the dose
continue to observe the patient in the coronary care unit

Fig. 14.5 Acute management of acute MI. (IV, intravenous; rt-PA, recombinant tissue plasminogen activator.)

trial and the International Study of Infarct Survival (ISIS) II study. This is because thrombolysis results in recanalization of the occluded vessel and restores coronary flow, which reduces infarct size and improves myocardial function if thrombolysis is administered within 24 hours of pain.

Thrombolytic agents

There are a number of thrombolytic agents (Fig. 14.6). The two most commonly used are streptokinase and recombinant tissue plasminogen activator (rt-PA). There are, however, an increasing number of new agents.

Two major trials GISSI II and ISIS 3 showed no increased benefit when comparing different thrombolytic agents—GISSI II streptokinase and t-PA; ISIS 3 streptokinase, rt-PA, and anisoylated plasminogen streptokinase activator complex (APSAC). These trials also showed that heparin provided no benefit. However, GUSTO (Global Use of Strategies to Open Occluded Arteries) 1 showed a small benefit with accelerated rt-PA followed by a heparin infusion over other regimens.

Contraindications to thrombolysis

All final year students and junior doctors must know this list:
- History of haemorrhagic cerebrovascular event ever.
- History of any type of cerebrovascular event in past 6 months.
- Recent gastrointestinal bleed.
- Bleeding diathesis or warfarin therapy with an International Normalized Ratio over 1.5.

- Operation within past month—not an absolute contraindication, but you should consult a senior before proceeding.
- Pregnancy.
- Any other invasive procedure in the past month (e.g. organ biopsy, dental extraction)—consult a senior before proceeding.

Indications for thrombolysis

Most centres consider a door to needle time of greater than 30 min unacceptable. Ideally all patients should be thrombolysed within 70 min of onset of pain to receive the greatest benefit.

All patients who satisfy the following criteria should be thrombolysed as soon as possible.
- History of chest pain lasting less than 24 hours.
- And one of the following—ST elevation greater than 1 mm in standard leads or in two adjacent chest leads or new bundle branch block on ECG.

Other agents used for acute myocardial infarction
Aspirin

The antiplatelet aggregation action of aspirin makes it effective in all acute coronary syndromes where the primary event is clot formation. This drug has relatively few side effects and should be administered promptly to all patients as soon as the ECG is found to be positive.

Aspirin was found to reduce the mortality rate in the ISIS II study.

Overview of thrombolytic agents				
Agent	Action	Half-life (min)	Administration	Other features
streptokinase	binds to plasminogen to form a complex that activates to convert another molecule of plasminogen to plasmin; not clot specific —will attack all plasminogen	18 (but 180 for streptokinase plasminogen complex)	infusion of 1.5 million units over 1 hour	allergic reactions, hypotension, previous streptokinase treatment renders subsequent doses less effective due to antibody production, haemorrhage
rt-PA	binds to fibrin and complex converts plasminogen to plasmin; clot specific—will only act in presence of fibrin	4–5 (circulating plasminogen and fibrinogen levels return to 80% of normal within 24 hours	infusion, often preceded by a bolus dose; accelerated t-PA—15 mg bolus then 50 mg over 30 min followed by 35 mg over 1 hour (as in the GUSTO trial)	haemorrhage, very expensive
APSAC	a stable form of the streptokinase–plasminogen complex that is activated in injection	long—100 min —therefore can be given as a single dose; enables the drug to be used in the community and can therefore be administered earlier	30 units intravenously	hypotension, haemorrhage, very expensive
the ideal thrombolytic agent	very clot specific, easily reversible in the event of haemorrhage; administration by intravenous bolus	very short half-life for use in hospital as infusion (can be easily controlled) and long half-life preparation for community use where coronary care not easily accessible		cheap, no antibody effects, derived from human protein so no anaphylaxis

Fig. 14.6 Overview of thrombolytic agents. (APSAC, anisoylated plasminogen streptokinase activator complex; rt-PA, recombinant tissue plasminogen activator.)

Diamorphine

A powerful anxiolytic and analgesic this drug is extremely effective in the patient who has cardiac pain. It has venodilating properties and is therefore also an effective antifailure agent.

β-blockers ((β-adrenoceptor antagonists)

These drugs were shown to reduce mortality rate acutely after MI in ISIS 1. The following are contraindications to the administration of β-blockers:
- Unstable or acute cardiac failure.
- Bradycardia (heart rate <60 beats/min).
- Hypotension (systolic blood pressure <90 mmHg).
- Asthma.

Oxygen

Oxygen should be administered to all patients initially and then continued for all patients who have hypoxaemia (i.e. arterial oxygen saturation <90%).

Non-acute management

The first 5–7 days after MI are spent in hospital because this is when most complications (Fig. 14.7) will arise.

The following points of management must be observed. The patient must be seen and examined every day by a cardiologist. Particular points to look for on examination and questioning are:
- Chest pain—further pain indicates the possibility of another MI and should be investigated early with urgent coronary angiogram.
- Breathlessness or signs of cardiac failure—diuretics should be commenced and urgent echocardiography performed to exclude septal defect or mitral regurgitation secondary to papillary muscle rupture.
- New murmurs—a ruptured papillary muscle causes mitral regurgitation; a ruptured septum causes ventricular septal defect.
- Pericardial rub—pericarditis.

109

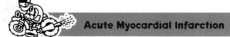

- Hypotension—drug induced or secondary to cardiogenic shock.
- Bradycardia—heart block after an inferior (or very large anterior MI with septal necrosis).

The patient should have daily ECGs to look for arrhythmias including heart block.

A continuous cardiac monitor should be used for the first 5 days because fatal arrhythmias are common after MI (usually ventricular tachycardia or fibrillation).

Early mobilization (after 48 hours) is instituted to prevent venous stasis.

If the patient has had a large MI or there is clinical evidence of cardiac failure (and provided there is no renal failure or hypotension) an angiotensin-converting enzyme inhibitor should be introduced at day 3 after MI. This improves outcome as seen in the ISIS 4 and GISSI 3 studies.

Hypercholesterolaemia should be treated with a statin and the patient referred to a lipid management clinic for follow-up. Suitable dietary advice should be given. Recent evidence suggests that a statin should be given any way because they may have additional benefits after MI in addition to their lipid lowering effect. The LIPID (Long-term Intervention with Pravastatin in Ischaemic Heart Disease) study shows benefit with pravastatin in patients after MI who have total cholesterol before treatment as low as 4.0 mmol/L.

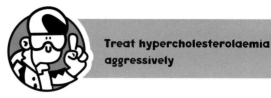
Treat hypercholesterolaemia aggressively

Follow-up care should include:
- An exercise test at about 6 weeks after MI to assess the risk of further ischaemia—if positive a coronary angiogram should be performed.
- Access to the rehabilitation programme.

Cardiac rehabilitation

All good cardiac units have an integrated rehabilitation programme available to all cardiac patients that consists of:
- Progressively increasing exercise level to a maintenance level of as much regular rapid walking as possible every day.
- Dietary advice, particularly emphasizing the value of fish and olive oil, and fresh fruit and vegetables. Carbohydrate restriction for non-insulin-dependent diabetes mellitus and insulin resistance. Calorie restriction for patients who have diabetes mellitus or who are obese.
- Advice on medications (Fig. 14.8), their role in improving prognosis, and the importance of compliance.
- Advice from a clinical psychologist on how to cope with the illness.

Complications of an AMI
Early (0–48 hours)
arrhythmias—VT, VF, SVT, heart block cardiogenic shock due to left or right ventricular failure
Medium term (2–7 days)

arrhythmias—VT,VF, SVT, heart block
pulmonary embolus (4–7 days)
rupture of papillary muscle (3–5 days)
rupture of interventricular septum (3–5 days)
free wall rupture (3–5 days)
(rupture of the above structures usually presents with acute
   cardiac failure and progresses rapidly to death; a few
   patients may survive after surgery)

Late (> 7 days)
arrhythmias—VT, VF, SVT, heart block cardiac failure Dressler's syndrome (3–8 weeks) left ventricular aneurysm (after several weeks) mural thrombosis and sytemic embolization

Fig. 14.7 Complications of an acute MI. (SVT, supraventricular tachycardia; VF, ventricular fibrillation; VT, ventricular tachycardia.)

Drugs on discharge after MI
aspirin
β-blocker
ACE inhibitor
a statin lipid-lowering drug—this should probably be given regardless of lipid levels as they seem to modify the progress of atheroma independently

Fig 14.8 Drugs on discharge after MI. (ACE, angiotensin-converting enzyme.)

- Group gymnasium sessions may help some patients by encouraging exercise and giving psychological support to each other.
- A subsequent support group may be continued as long as each individual patient finds it helpful; a doctor's input is important from time to time.

SUMMARY OF MANAGEMENT OF ISCHAEMIC CHEST PAIN

An algorithm summarizing the management of ischaemic chest pain is given in Fig. 14.9.

HEART BLOCK AFTER MYOCARDIAL INFARCTION

Ischaemic injury may occur at any point in the conducting system whether it be the sinoatrial node or the atrioventricular node or anywhere from the Bundle of His downwards.

It is therefore not surprising that heart block after MI may be:

- First or second degree atrioventricular block.
- Complete heart block with atrioventricular dissociation.
- Interventricular block (complete or partial RBBB or LBBB).

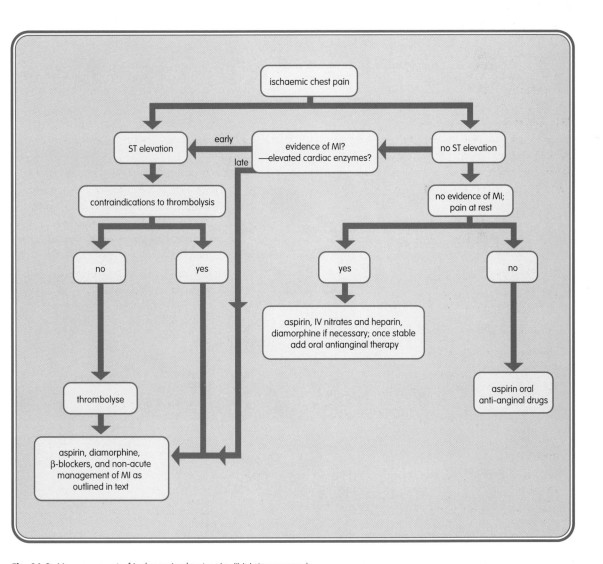

Fig. 14.9 Management of ischaemic chest pain. (IV, intravenous.)

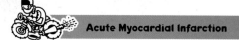

Inferior MI is more commonly associated with atrioventricular block because the atrioventricular node is supplied by the right coronary artery in 90% of cases.

Anterior MI may cause heart block if there is marked septal necrosis (indicating a large anterior MI).

Management of post-myocardial infarction heart block

Patients who have Mobitz type II or complete heart block should have temporary pacing wires inserted as soon as possible.

The need for a permanent pacemaker depends upon the site of the MI.

Patients who have anterior MI and septal necrosis often need permanent pacing because the atrioventricular node rarely recovers.

Patients who have an inferior MI may not need permanent pacing because many recover normal function of the atrioventricular node. Current practice is to wait at least 2 weeks before deciding on a permanent system because recovery can take up to 3 weeks.

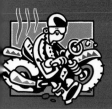

15. Supraventricular Tachyarrhythmias

DEFINITION OF SUPRAVENTRICULAR TACHYARRHYTHMIAS

Supraventricular tachyarrhythmias (SVTs) are fast rhythms characterized by narrow QRS complexes (unless abberrant conduction is present).

A tachycardia is defined as a rate of 100 beats/min or greater. In ascending order of atrial electrical dysfunction, these are:
- Sinus tachycardia.
- Atrial ectopics.
- Nodal ectopics.
- Atrial tachycardia.
- Junctional tachycardia and supraventricular re-entry tachycardia.
- Atrial flutter.
- Atrial fibrillation.

SINUS TACHYCARDIA

Points of importance are:
- The sinus node fires at over 100 beats/min.
- Every complex is preceded by a normal P wave.
- The PR interval is within normal limits and remains stable.

Causes
Causes of sinus tachycardia include:
- Fever.
- Thyrotoxicosis.
- Hypotension.
- Any form of stress (e.g. pain, anxiety, exertion).

These are all physiological responses. Rarely an inappropriate resting sinus tachycardia occurs. This is due to an abnormality of sinus node discharge or another atrial focus of activity located near the sinus node.

PREMATURE ATRIAL ECTOPICS

These are seen on the ECG as a premature P wave (which may be normal or abnormal in appearance) followed by a prolonged PR interval (>120 ms). They are followed by a pause because the atrioventricular (AV) node is refractory.

Premature atrial ectopics can be precipitated by many conditions including:
- Stress.
- Caffeine.
- Alcohol.
- Myocardial ischaemia.
- Myocardial inflammation.

Treatment is not indicated unless the patient is very symptomatic in which case β-blockers (β-adrenoceptor antagonists) may be of some help.

NODAL AND JUNCTIONAL ECTOPICS

The AV node is a compact structure and lying close to it is the AV junctional area. It is from this area and from the node itself that these ectopic beats originate. These structures have the ability to fire autonomously, but they have a slower rate of firing than the sinoatrial (SA) node therefore they are usually suppressed.

In some conditions impulses may arise ectopically from the AV node and junctional region.

The impulse is conducted to the atrium where a retrograde P wave is produced and also to the ventricle where a narrow complex QRS is produced (Fig.15.1). (Depending upon the speed of conduction the P wave may occur just before, after, or simultaneously with the QRS.)

Again treatment is not usually indicated.

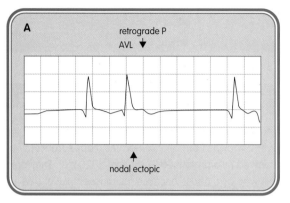

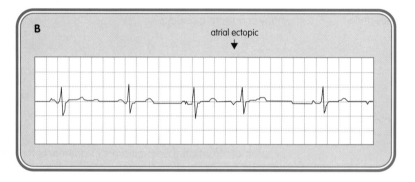

Fig. 15.1 (A) A nodal ectopic. The ectopic complex is similar to the normal QRS suggesting that it originates from the atrioventricular or junctional region. The P wave is retrograde and is seen just after the ectopic QRS superimposed on the T wave. The ectopic beat is followed by a compensatory pause. **(B)** ECG illustrating an ectopic atrial beat. Note that the premature atrial beat fires an abnormally shaped P wave and a normal QRS complex. A compensatory pause follows.

ATRIAL TACHYCARDIA

Atrial tachycardia is a tachyarrhythmia generated in the atrial tissue. The atrial rate is 150–200 beats/min.

Because the origin of the tachycardia is not the SA node the P wave morphology is different to normal. The P wave axis may also be abnormal, for example, when the atrial focus is in the left atrium the P wave in lead V1 is positive.

Causes
The following may lead to atrial tachycardia:
- Structural heart abnormality.
- Coronary artery disease.
- Digitalis toxicity.

Investigation and diagnosis
On examination the pulse is rapid and of variable intensity:
- Jugular venous pressure may reveal many a waves to each v wave if there is a degree of AV block.
- ECG may show 1:1 conduction or variable degrees of AV block.

- It may be difficult to differentiate atrial tachycardia from atrial flutter.

Diagnosis may be aided by enhancing AV block and therefore making it easier to visualize the P wave morphology and rate. There are two effective methods of doing this:
- Carotid sinus massage—increases vagal stimulation of the SA and AV node.
- Intravenous adenosine—results in transient complete AV block.

Remember that atrial flutter usually has an atrial rate of 300/min with a degree of AV block. Atrial tachycardia has a slightly slower atrial rate with abnormal P waves.

Management
The patient will present with palpitations. Any underlying cause should be treated (e.g. check digoxin levels and stop the drug).

Drugs used to treat atrial tachycardia include:
- Atrioventricular blocking drugs such as digoxin, β-blockers (β-adrenoceptor antagonists), calcium channel blockers—these slow the ventricular response rate, but do not affect the atrial tachycardia itself).
- Class 1A (e.g. disopyramide), 1C (e.g. flecainide), or III (e.g. amiodarone) drugs (see p. 121) may be used to try and terminate the atrial tachycardia.

Electrical cardioversion is often successful.

ATRIOVENTRICULAR JUNCTIONAL TACHYCARDIA

Tachycardias arising from the junctional area occur when there is a focus of activity with a discharge rate that is faster than that of the SA node. This is an abnormal situation and is usually due to ischaemic heart disease or digitalis toxicity.

Clinical features
The following features are seen
- Rate is usually up to 130 beats/min.
- Gradual onset.
- Terminates gradually.
- ECG shows a narrow complex tachycardia occasionally with retrogradely conducted P waves. It is difficult to distinguish this from an AV nodal re-entry tachycardia and you will not be expected to do so. The main point is to realise that the junctional tissue may be a site of ectopic electrical activity.

Management
Treatment is aimed at the underlying cause:
- Antiarrhythmic agents such as digoxin, β-blockers, and calcium channel antagonists may be tried.
- Electrical cardioversion may be successful.

ATRIOVENTRICULAR NODAL RE-ENTRANT TACHYCARDIA

These tachycardias involve a re-entry circuit that lies in or close to the AV node and allows impulses to travel round and round triggering the ventricles and the atria (in a retrograde manner) as they go.

Clinical features
These tachycardias display the following features:
- Rate is 150–260 beats/min.
- Usually sudden onset and offset.
- QRS complexes are narrow unless there is aberrant conduction and the P waves may occur just before, just after, or within the QRS (it is not always easy to see these) (see Fig. 4.3C).

Causes of re-entrant tachycardia are caffeine, alcohol and anxiety.

Diagnosis
Differentiation from atrial flutter and atrial fibrillation (AF) can be made by either:
- Performing carotid sinus massage or Valsalva manoeuvre.
- Giving intravenous adenosine.

These procedures block the AV node and therefore the P waves of atrial flutter can be seen or the baseline fibrillation of AF can be seen. Blockade of the AV node in re-entrant tachycardia breaks the re-entry circuit and terminates the tachycardia in most cases.

Management
These tachycardias often terminate spontaneously with relaxation.

Vagal manoeuvres such as carotid sinus massage and the Valsalva manoeuvre are often effective in terminating the tachycardia and patients can be taught to do these themselves.

In hospital the following treatments can be effective:
- Vagal manoeuvres.
- Intravenous adenosine.
- Atrioventricular node blocking agents (e.g. β-blockers, digoxin, calcium channel blockers).
- Direct current (DC) cardioversion if less invasive methods have been unsuccessful.

In a patient who has recurrent troublesome AV nodal re-entry tachycardia electrophysiological testing can locate the site of the abnormal circuit and this can then be ablated. This is a curative procedure. The main risk is AV node ablation resulting in complete heart block and requiring a permanent pacemaker.

115

WOLFF–PARKINSON–WHITE SYNDROME

In this condition there is an abnormal connection between the atrium and the ventricle along, which the impulse can travel. This is known as an accessory pathway. In Wolff–Parkinson–White syndrome the accessory pathway is known as the bundle of Kent.

Characteristics of the bundle of Kent

The bundle of Kent is capable of:

- Anterograde conduction—that is it can conduct from the atrium to the ventricle; it is also capable of retrograde conduction.
- Conducting impulses faster than the normal His conductive tissue. Therefore the ventricle is activated sooner than normal.

If, however, the impulse does not travel down the bundle of Kent, the P wave and QRS complex are normal. Therefore it can be seen that the impulse can travel via two different routes from the atrium to the ventricle.

The impulse often travels both routes simultaneously; this results in a short PR interval and a slurred upstroke to the R wave (known as a delta wave; Fig. 15.2).

Tachycardias associated with Wolff–Parkinson–White syndrome

A number of tachycardias may occur:

- Atrioventricular re-entry tachycardia—the impulse is conducted from the atrium to the ventricle via the AV node then back to the atrium via the accessory pathway—this results in a narrow complex tachycardia.
- A similar tachycardia with conduction in the opposite direction (i.e. from the atrium to the ventricle via the accessory pathway) results in a broad complex tachycardia because the ventricle is depolarized from a point away from the bundle of His.
- Atrial fibrillation and atrial flutter may occur and may present a potential risk because the atrial impulses can be conducted rapidly via the accessory pathway giving ventricular rates of 300 beats/min or greater. This rapid ventricular rate predisposes to ventricular fibrillation.

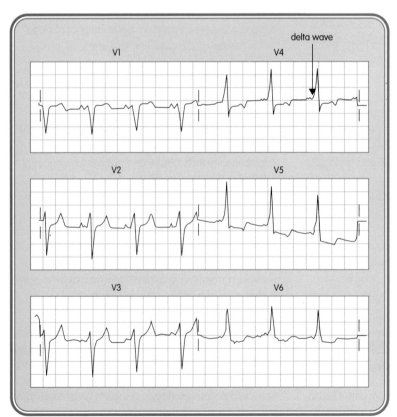

Fig. 15.2 Wolff–Parkinson–White syndrome. Note the short PR interval (<0.08 s) and the slurred upstroke of the QRS complex (the delta wave).This is caused by part of the impulse travelling down the accessory pathway and causing pre-excitation (early excitation) of the ventricle (represented by the delta wave). The rest of the impulse travels via the atrioventricular node and is represented by the main QRS complex.

Clinical features

Wolff–Parkinson–White syndrome is a congenital condition. Patients present with recurrent palpitations or syncope. Sudden death is a risk due to ventricular tachycardia. The accessory pathway may cease to conduct as patients grow older, but other patients continue to have problems.

Management

Treatment of Wolff–Parkinson–White syndrome is indicated only in patients who have recurrent tachyarrhythmias; some patients have ECG evidence of the accessory pathway (short PR and delta wave), but no tachyarrhythmia and these do not require treatment.

There are a number of treatment options; the main ones to consider are drug therapy and ablation therapy.

Drug therapy

The aim of drug therapy is to slow conduction in the accessory pathway as well as to slow AV conduction. Drugs that do both are Vaughan Williams classification IA, IC, and III drugs (see p. 121).

Drugs such as digoxin and verapamil block the AV node, but do not affect the accessory pathway, so increasing the risk of rapid conduction of AF and flutter via the accessory pathway.

So remember that digoxin and verapamil should not be used as single agents in the treatment of tachycardias in Wolff–Parkinson–White syndrome.

Ablation therapy

This may be surgical or electrical:

- Electrical ablation (or radiofrequency catheter ablation) is performed after the accessory pathway has been located by electrophysiological testing. This procedure is usually performed under light sedation using local anaesthetic before inserting the electrodes.
- Surgical ablation is rarely performed, but may be useful if electrical ablation is not successful.

ATRIAL FLUTTER

Atrial flutter has the following characteristics:

- Atrial contraction rate is regular and is 250–350 beats/min (usually 300 beats/min).
- Ventricular response may be 1:1 (300 beats/min), 2:1 (150 beats/min), 3:1 (100 beats/min), etc.

- Severity of the symptoms depends upon the ventricular response rate (i.e. a rapid ventricular response is likely to cause palpitations, angina, and cardiac failure).

Causes include:

- Structural heart disease (e.g. valve disease, cardiomyopathy).
- Pulmonary disease (e.g. pulmonary embolus, pneumothorax, infection).
- Toxins (e.g. alcohol, caffeine).

Investigations and diagnosis

The ECG findings are (Fig. 15.3):

- Regular sawtooth atrial flutter waves (P waves).
- Narrow QRS complexes (unless there is coexistent bundle branch block).

Diagnosis is confirmed by performing AV nodal blocking manoeuvres (e.g. adenosine or carotid sinus massage). This slows the ventricular response so that the sawtooth P waves are revealed on the ECG.

Management

Cardioversion back to sinus rhythm is the best treatment, but if this is not possible then slowing of the ventricular rate will provide symptomatic relief and protect against cardiac failure. Direct current cardioversion using a synchronized shock will rapidly and safely restore sinus rhythm in some cases. Class IA, IC or III drugs (see p. 121) may be useful:

- Where DC cardioversion is unsuccessful to chemically cardiovert to sinus rhythm.
- To maintain sinus rhythm after successful electrical cardioversion.

Where cardioversion is not possible or not sustained AV blocking agents are used to slow the ventricular response rate (class II, class IV, or digoxin).

There is an increased risk of thrombus formation in atrial flutter so anticoagulation is recommended before DC cardioversion, as with atrial fibrillation.

ATRIAL FIBRILLATION

Atrial fibrillation has the following features:

- It is a common arrhythmia found in over 55% of the population over 70 years of age.

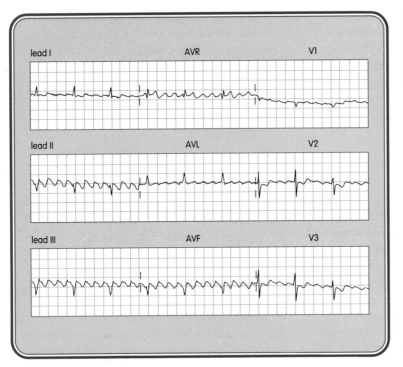

Fig. 15.3 Atrial flutter. Note the sawtooth F waves at a rate of just over 300 beats/min and the ventricular response of 4:1. Leads II and V1 often show P waves best (but not in this case).

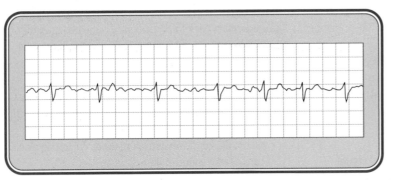

Fig. 15.4 Atrial fibrillation. Note the irregular baseline and the lack of P waves. The rhythm is irregularly irregular.

- There is disorganized random electrical activity in the atria resulting in a lack of effective atrial contraction.
- Stasis of blood in the atria predisposes to thrombus formation and embolic episodes.

Causes

Common causes are as follows:
- Ischaemic heart disease.
- Valvular heart disease, especially mitral valve disease.
- Hypertensive heart disease.
- Pulmonary disease (e.g. embolus, infection, pneumothorax).
- Any form of sepsis.
- Thyrotoxicosis.
- Alcohol excess.

Investigations and diagnosis

The ECG shows no P waves and an irregular baseline with a variable ventricular response rate (hence the irregularly irregular pulse; Fig. 15.4). Ventricular response ranges from 90 to 170 beats/min, but can be faster or slower. The actual AF rate may be from 300 to 600 beats/min. Because of the absence of atrial contraction there are no a waves in the jugular venous pressure waveform and no fourth heart sound.

Management

The likelihood of successful cardioversion depends upon:
- Persistence of the underlying cause (e.g. a patient who has untreated mitral stenosis is unlikely to cardiovert successfully whereas a patient who has angina treated with medication or angioplasty is).
- Duration of the AF (i.e. the longer the duration the smaller the chance of cardioversion).

Treatment options are similar to those of atrial flutter:
- DC cardioversion (often requiring higher energy than for atrial flutter) may cardiovert the patient into sinus rhythm.
- Pharmacological agents from groups IA, IC and III (see p. 121) can be used to cardiovert or to maintain sinus rhythm after electrical cardioversion.
- Patients who have resistant AF may be treated with an AV node blocking agent to slow the electrical response (group II or IV drugs or digoxin).

Anticoagulation and atrial fibrillation

Atrial fibrillation carries an increased risk of thromboembolism because of cerebrovascular and peripheral embolization in particular. Benefits of anticoagulation must be balanced against risk of haemorrhage before the decision to anticoagulate is made. The following points must be recognized:
- Patients who have structural heart disease (e.g. valve lesion, dilated left ventricle) and AF have a higher risk of thromboembolic complications than those who have lone AF (i.e. AF with no obvious underlying cause).
- Patients who have other risk factors for thromboembolism (e.g. hypertension, diabetes mellitus, previous cerebral embolus) have a higher risk of thromboembolism.
- Older patients who have AF are at a greater risk.
- Warfarin reduces the risk of cerebral embolus by approximately 60–80%.
- Aspirin reduces the risk of cerebral embolus by approximately 40%.

The following are possible guidelines for the use of anticoagulation in patients who have AF:
- Patients under 60 years of age who have no structural heart disease and no other risk factors are treated with aspirin alone because the risk of thromboembolism is approximately 1% and does not justify the risk of warfarinization.
- Any patient over 60 years of age and all patients regardless of age who have structural heart disease or additional rsk factors should be anticoagulated with warfarin unless there are any contraindications.
- Anticoagulation should be carefully monitored especially in the elderly. As mentioned above this group of patients have a higher risk of haemorrhage with anticoagulation). The International Normalized Ratio (INR) should be maintained at between 2 and 3.

Anticoagulation and cardioversion of AF

There is an increased risk of thromboembolism after cardioversion of AF to sinus rhythm. This is thought to be due to the formation of atrial thrombus before cardioversion and the persistence of inefficient contraction in certain parts of the atrium (e.g. left atrial appendage) for a few weeks after apparently successful cardioversion. Therefore there is a risk of intracardiac clot forming for a few weeks, even after successful cardioversion. Points to note are as follows:
- If the AF is of recent onset (within 48–72 hours) it is reasonable to anticoagulate the patient with intravenous heparin and cardiovert straight away.
- If the patient has a longer history full anticoagulation should be given (warfarin with an INR 2–3) for at least 4 weeks before cardioversion and continued for 1 month after cardioversion.
- In patients where emergency cardioversion is required (i.e. patients who have severe heart failure secondary to AF) cardioversion should be performed with heparin cover immediately.
- Transoesophageal echocardiography is a reliable way of excluding intracardiac clot and can be used to see whether it is safe to proceed to cardioversion immediately in an unanticoagulated patient

INVESTIGATION OF PATIENTS WHO HAVE SUPRAVENTRICULAR TACHYARRHYTHMIAS

The following investigations are appropriate for all patients who have an SVT.

Blood tests

These include:
- Electrolytes—hypokalaemia may predispose to tachyarrhythmias and also to digoxin toxicity.
- Thyroid function tests.

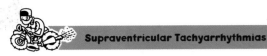

- Full blood count—anaemia may precipitate ischaemia.
- Liver function tests, particularly γ-glutamyltransferase, which is abnormal in patients who have excess alcohol intake.

Electrocardiography

Features that may be evident include:
- The arrhythmia.
- Ischaemic changes—these are usually accentuated during a tachycardia due to increased cardiac oxygen demand.
- Hypertensive changes.
- Pre-excitation.

24- or 48-hour electrocardiography

This may be useful in identifying paroxysmal tachyarrhythmias.

Chest radiography

Notable features may include:
- Cardiomegaly or pulmonary oedema.
- Valve calcification.

Echocardiography

This may be useful because:
- Valve lesions and dilated cardiac chambers may be identified.
- Transoesophageal echocardiography will exclude intracardiac clot.

Electrophysiological studies

These are useful for arrhythmias when it is difficult to identify the mechanism and any possible focus or accessory pathway suitable for ablation.

Atrioventricular nodal blocking manoeuvres

These are used diagnostically and therapeutically:
- Diagnostically—they slow the ventricular response and enable P wave morphology to be seen.
- Therapeutically—they are used to terminate arrhythmias with re-entry circuits involving the AV node.

The following manoeuvres are appropriate:
- Carotid sinus massage.
- Valsalva manoeuvre—straining against a closed glottis.
- Adenosine administration (rapid intravenous injection).

Carotid sinus massage

This increases vagal tone and so prolongs AV node conduction time. The patient should be lying comfortably with the neck extended. Carotid bruits must be excluded (carotid artery occlusion may cause a stroke if the opposite side is heavily diseased).

The patient should preferably be connected to a 12-lead ECG running all 12 leads simultaneously. If only a few leads are running the P waves may not be seen.

Initial gentle and then firm pressure is applied to the carotid pulse just below the angle of the jaw. Remember—never do this on both sides simultaneously.

Pressure is applied for a maximum of 5–10 s.

Adenosine administration

Again the patient should be supine and connected to a 12-lead ECG continuous trace. Warn the patient that he or she may experience chest pain, flushing, and dyspnoea for a few seconds after administration.

Establish intravenous access in a good-sized vein (antecubital fossa is ideal). Start with 3 mg rapid intravenous injection, follow with a rapid normal saline flush of 20 ml. If there is no response this may be repeated with incrementally higher doses up to 18 mg.

Actions of adenosine

Adenosine activates potassium channels and hyperpolarizes the cell menbrane. It acts to slow AV conduction time

The half-life of adenosine is very short (6 s) and it can be safely used to differentiate ventricular tachycardia from SVT with aberrant conduction. After adenosine the P waves will be revealed in SVT or the SVT may be terminated.

If verapamil is used for this purpose there is a risk of fatal myocardial depression in patients who have ventricular tachycardia.

Adenosine may precipitate bronchospasm and should be avoided in asthmatic patients.

DRUGS USED TO TREAT TACHYARRHYTHMIAS

The older Vaughan Williams classification is still sometimes used:

- Class I—inhibitors of sodium current (i.e. local anaesthetic like).
- Class II—β-adrenergic receptor antagonists.
- Class III—inhibitors of repolarization, which prolong the action potential and refractory period.
- Class IV—inhibitors of calcium current.
- Digitalis glycosides.

A summary of the electrophysiological actions of antiarrhythmic drugs is given in Fig. 15.5. It can be seen from this that class 1A, 1C, and III drugs affect conduction in the atrial and ventricular tissue—they are therefore useful for cardioverting many rhythms to sinus by breaking re-entry circuits or reducing the excitability of ectopic foci. Class III drugs have the added advantage of slowing AV conduction and therefore slowing ventricular response as well.

Class II and IV drugs and digoxin act as AV node blockers. This is useful in slowing the ventricular response and will cardiovert rhythms that are caused by re-entry circuits involving the AV node (e.g. AV nodal re-entry tachycardias and AV re-entry tachycardias).

A summary of the pharmacokinetics and side effects of antiarrhythmic agents is shown in Fig. 15.6.

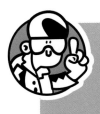

All antiarrhythmic agents can cause bradyarrhythmias and extreme caution should be exercised when using them in combination.

Electrophysiological actions of antiarrhythmic drugs						
Vaughan Williams class of drug	Examples	Site of action	Sinus node rate	Atrial conduction rate	AV node refractory period	Ventricular conduction rate
IA	quinidine, procainamide, disopyramide	block fast sodium channels	no effect	decreased	increased	decreased
IB	lignocaine, mexiletine, tocainide	block fast sodium channels	no effect	no effect	not much effect (may slightly increase or decrease)	decreased
IC	flecainide, propafenone	block fast sodium channels	reduced	decreased	increased	decreased
II	atenolol, metoprolol, sotalol, propanolol	block β-adrenergic receptors	reduced	no effect	increased	no effect
III	amiodarone, sotalol, bretylium	block potassium channels; mechanism not entirely understood	reduced	decreased	increased	decreased
IV	verapamil, diltiazem	block slow calcium channels	small reduction	slightly reduced	increased	no effect
digoxin	blocks Na/K ATPase	no effect	no effect	increased	no effect; ? slows AV conduction	? slows AV conduction

Fig. 15.5 Electrophysiological actions of antiarrhythmic drugs.

Pharmacokinetics and adverse effects of antiarrhythmic drugs					
Drug	Route of administration	Half-life	Mode of excretion	Interactions	Adverse effects
procainamide	oral, IV, or IM	3–5 hours	renal	amiodarone reduces clearance	skin rashes, Raynaud' syndrome, hallucinations; toxicity—cardiac failure, long QT, ventricular tachyarrhythmias
lignocaine	IV (extensive first pass metabolism in liver)	1–2 hours	hepatic	cimetidine reduces clearance	myocardial depression, cardiac failure, long QT; toxicity—dizziness, confusion, paraesthesia
flecainide	oral, IV	20 hours	renal (partly hepatic)	cimetidine reduces clearance	myocardial depression, ventricular arrhythmias (a major problem, especially in patients who have ischaemic heart disease)
atenolol	oral, IV		renal	may precipitate asthma or peripheral ischaemia	myocardial depression, bronchospasm, peripheral vasoconstriction
sotalol	oral, IV	10–15 hours	renal	may precipitate asthma or peripheral ischaemia	myocardial depression, long QT, ventricular tachyarrhythmias
amiodarone	oral, IV	3–6 weeks	hepatic	reduces digoxin excretion, reduces warfarin excretion (need to watch INR closely)	pulmonary fibrosis, liver damage, peripheral neuropathy, hyper- or hypothyroidism, corneal microdeposits, photosensitivity, myocardial depression (but safe in cardiac failure), long QT
verapamil	oral, IV	3–7 hours	renal	reduces digoxin excretion	myocardial depression, constipation
digoxin	oral, IV	36–48 hours	renal	amiodarone, verapamil, and propafenone decrease renal clearance; erythromycin increases absorption; captopril decreases renal clearance	toxicity—heart block, atrial tachycardia, ventricular arrhythmia, xanthopsia

Fig. 15.6 Pharmacokinetics and adverse effects of antiarrhythmic drugs. Note that a common complication of all antiarrhythmic agents is bradycardia, which may be severe. Care must always be used when increasing dosage or combining more than one agent. (IM, intramuscular; INR, international normalized ratio; IV, intravenous.)

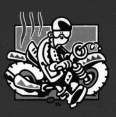

16. Ventricular Tachyarrhythmias

DEFINITION OF VENTRICULAR TACHYARRHYTHMIAS

A ventricular tachyarrhythmia is an abnormal rapid rhythm that originates in the ventricular myocardium or the His–Purkinje system.

Ventricular tachyarrhythmias are broad complex —the QRS complex is greater than 0.12 s in duration or three small squares on a standard ECG trace.

There are four basic types of ventricular tachyarrhythmia:
- Ventricular ectopic beats.
- Ventricular tachycardia.
- Torsades de pointes.
- Ventricular fibrillation.

VENTRICULAR ECTOPIC BEATS

Also known as ventricular premature beats, these beats have certain ECG characteristics (Fig. 16.1) such as:
- They occur before the next normal beat would be due.
- They are not preceded by a P wave.
- The QRS complex is abnormal in shape and has a duration of greater than 120 ms.
- They are followed by a compensatory pause so that the RR interval between the normal beats immediately preceding and immediately following the ectopic beat is exactly twice the normal RR interval.

Clinical features

It is thought that ventricular ectopics occur in over half the normal population. This prevalence increases with age. These extra beats do not necessarily imply underlying heart disease.

Most people are entirely asymptomatic; others may complain of missed or extra beats. Alternatively others may experience thumping or heavy beats because the beat immediately following the ectopic does so after a compensatory pause during which there is a prolonged filling time resulting in an increased stroke volume plus post-extrasystolic potentiation of contractility.

A number of precipitating causes of ventricular premature beats are recognized including:
- Low serum potassium.
- Excess caffeine consumption.
- Febrile illness.
- Underlying cardiac abnormality (e.g. recent myocardial infarction, cardiomyopathy, mitral or aortic valve disease).

Management

The clinical significance of ventricular ectopic beats is unclear and the general rule is that in a patient who has no underlying cardiac abnormality no treatment is needed unless symptoms are severe (in this situation a small dose of β-blocker should suppress ectopic activity).

In the post-myocardial infarction situation there is currently much controversy regarding the significance

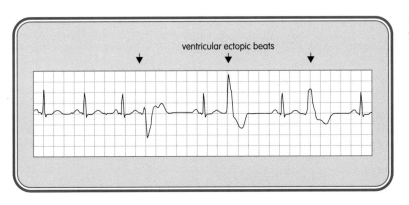

Fig. 16.1 Ventricular ectopic beats, which are indicated by arrows.

of, and need to treat, ventricular ectopics. There is no evidence currently that treatment of ventricular premature beats after myocardial infarction reduces mortality rate. Current opinion therefore seems to be that provided that hypokalaemia is treated no antiarrhythmic agents are indicated to treat ventricular premature beats in the post-myocardial infarction patient.

VENTRICULAR TACHYCARDIA

Ventricular tachycardia (VT) is defined as three or more consecutive ventricular beats occurring at a rate greater than 120 beats/min (Fig. 16.2). Again the complexes are abnormal and their duration is longer than 120 ms.

Clinical features

Patients occasionally tolerate this rhythm well and experience only palpitations or rarely nothing at all.

More commonly the reduction in cardiac output caused by this arrhythmia causes dizziness or syncope.

Common precipitants include hypokalaemia and acute myocardial infarction.

Diagnosis

The main differential diagnosis for VT is supraventricular tachycardia with aberrant conduction (or bundle branch block) (Fig. 16.3). This causes much confusion and concern amongst junior doctors and final year students alike. It helps if you remember the following points:

- Both arrhythmias are potentially fatal so treat each with respect.
- The use of carotid sinus massage or adenosine may briefly block the atrioventricular node and therefore slow the ventricular response in supraventricular tachycardia (it will have no effect on VT).
- Never use verapamil or lignocaine to slow the ventricular response in this situation: the negative inotropic effect of this drug could have disastrous effects if the rhythm is in fact VT causing rapid development of cardiac failure.

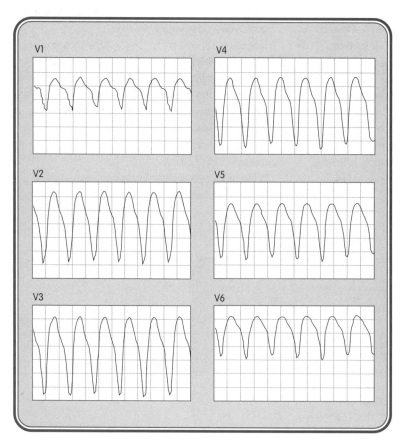

Fig. 16.2 ECG illustrating ventricular tachycardia. Note the concordance shown in the chest leads. No fusion or capture beats seen.

Management

Ventricular tachycardia is very dangerous and if allowed to continue will result in cardiac failure. Treatment must therefore be prompt and the nature of the treatment depends upon the clinical scenario.

- Patient conscious with intermittent episodes of VT—treatment should be with drugs (these are discussed on p. 127).
- Patient conscious with ongoing VT—triggered (synchronized) direct current (DC) cardioversion under general anaesthetic.
- Patient compromised and unconscious with ongoing VT—praecordial thump followed by triggered (synchronized) DC cardioversion according to resuscitation council guidelines (see Chapter 18).

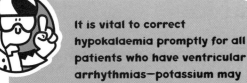

It is vital to correct hypokalaemia promptly for all patients who have ventricular arrhythmias—potassium may be given orally or in a very dilute form via a peripheral vein; in the emergency situation larger doses of potassium can be given via a central line with careful monitoring of cardiac rhythm and serum potassium levels. Warning: intravenous potassium can cause ventricular fibrillation.

VENTRICULAR FIBRILLATION

Ventricular fibrillation (VF) is irregular rapid ventricular depolarization (Fig. 16.4). There is no organized contraction of the ventricle, therefore the patient has no pulse. This arrhythmia rapidly causes loss of consciousness and cardiorespiratory arrest.

Clinical features

The most common cause of VF is acute myocardial infarction.

Ventricular fibrillation is also seen at the end-stage of many disease processes and signifies the presence of severe myocardial damage (this is sometimes referred to as secondary VF and usually results in death despite resuscitation attempts). It may be precipitated by:

- A ventricular ectopic beat.
- Ventricular tachycardia.
- Torsades de pointes.

Management

Ventricular fibrillation must be treated promptly with a praecordial thump and if this is unsuccessful with simple (non-synchronized) DC cardioversion (the resuscitation protocol is discussed in Chapter 17).

Antiarrhythmic agents are used prophylactically in certain patients who are at risk of recurrent episodes of VF. There is currently much debate about whether patients who have VF after myocardial infarction should be prophylactically treated with antiarrhythmic agents to

Differences between VT and SVT with BBB		
Arrhythmia	VT	SVT with BBB
QRS duration	>140 ms	not always
AV association	AV dissociation (no relationship between P waves and QRS)	P waves if seen are associated with the QRS
Variety of complexes	capture beats (where a P wave is followed by a normal QRS); fusion beats (where a normal sinus beat occurs simultaneously with a ventricular beat, the resulting complex having an intermediate appearance that is a combination of the two component beats)	no capture or fusion beats
ECG pattern	may be RBBB or LBBB	usually RBBB
Concordance	present (the QRS complexes retain the same axis throughout the chest leads)	absent (some QRS complexes will be positive, others will be negative)
QRS waveform	may vary from beat to beat	constant

Fig. 16.3 Differences between ventricular tachycardia (VT) and supraventricular tachycardia (SVT) with bundle branch block (BBB). (AV, atrioventricular; LBBB, left BBB; RBBB, right BBB.)

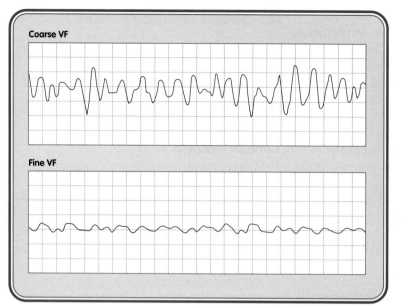

Fig. 16.4 Ventricular fibrillation (VF) may have a coarse or a fine pattern.

Coarse VF

Fine VF

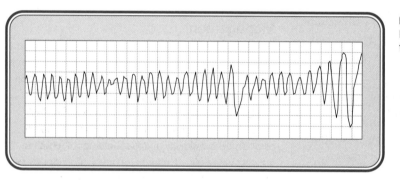

Fig. 16.5 Torsades de pointes. Note the irregular rhythm and twisting axis.

reduce mortality rate from subsequent ventricular arrhythmias; opinion is divided.

TORSADES DE POINTES

This rhythm is usually self-terminating, but can occasionally lead to VF and death. It is an irregular rapid rhythm with a characteristic twisting axis seen on the ECG (Fig. 16.5). In between episodes the ECG shows a long QT interval.

Clinical features

The patient usually feels faint or loses consciousness due to a drop in cardiac output. Attacks are much more likely to occur during periods of adrenergic stimulation (e.g. fear). There are many possible causes, all of which cause a prolonged QT interval (Fig. 16.6).

The QT interval corresponds to the time from depolarization to repolarization (beginning of the Q wave to end of T wave i.e. action potential duration, see *Crash Course: Cardiovascular System* by R. Sunthareswaran) and varies according to the heart rate. Therefore, a long QT interval is approximated by a corrected QT interval (QTc) of greater than 0.44 s. QTc = QT/square root of RR interval.

Fig. 16.6 Causes of long QT interval.

Causes of long QT interval	
Cause	**Examples**
congenital	Jervell and Lange–Nielsen syndrome (autosomal recessive and senorineural deafness) Romano–Ward syndrome (autosomal dominant, no deafness)
drugs	class 1A (e.g. quinidine, procainamide) class 3 (e.g. amiodarone, sotalol) tricyclic antidepressants (e.g. amitriptyline) phenothiazines (e.g. chlorpromazine) terfenadine
electrolyte abnormalities	hypokalaemia hypomagnesaemia hypocalcaemia
others	acute myocardial infarction central nervous system disease mitral valve prolapse organophosphate insecticides

Management

Treatment of torsades de pointes differs from that of the other ventricular arrhythmias and is as follows:

- Identify and treat any precipitating factors (stop offending drugs, correct electrolyte imbalance).
- Atrial or ventricular pacing to maintain a heart rate of no less than 90 beats/min to prevent lengthening of the QT interval—intravenous isoprenaline may also be used to reduce the QT interval.
- In congenital long QT syndromes high-dose β-blockers (β-adrenoceptor antagonists) or left stellectomy may be used and there is increasing use of permanent pacemakers and cardiovertor defibrillators.
- Do not use antiarrhythmic drugs.

DRUGS USED TO TREAT VENTRICULAR TACHYCARDIA AND FIBRILLATION

In the acute situation, if the patient is unconscious or has no cardiac output, a praecordial thump followed by DC cardioversion is used initially at 200 J. If the arrhythmia persists further resuscitation is carried out according to the set protocol. This is discussed in Chapter 17.

The drugs used to treat ventricular tachyarrhythmias other than torsades de pointes fall into two main classes:

- Class I.
- Class III.

In the acutely ill patient who has VT or VF, intravenous antiarrhythmic agents are given after sinus rhythm has been established by DC cardioversion (Fig. 16.7). These are given in the form of an infusion, usually in an attempt to stabilize the myocardium. Amiodarone, lignocaine, and flecainide are commonly used, but the latter two are dangerously negatively inotropic.

The exact drug chosen depends upon the individual. The following are some considerations worth noting:

- Amiodarone has many long-term side effects so caution must be used when prescribing it and the patient needs careful follow-up.
- Amiodarone is a good choice for the patient who has cardiac failure because it has been shown to be safe in heart failure.
- If given intravenously amiodarone must be given centrally because it is extremely damaging to peripheral veins.
- Amiodarone has a very long half-life (25 days) and oral loading takes at least 1 month. Intravenous loading is faster.
- In a patient who has no contraindication for β-blockers sotalol is a good long-term agent because it has none of the long-term side effects of amiodarone.

Class of agent	Class I	Class II	Class III	Class IV	Digoxin
Examples	IA—quinidine, procainamide, disopyramide; IB—lignocaine, mexiletine, tocainide; IC—flecainide, propafenone	β-blockers (e.g. atenolol, bisoprolol, metoprolol); sotalol also has some class III activity	amiodarone, sotalol, bretylium	calcium channel blockers (e.g. diltiazem, verapamil)	not classified by the Vaughan Williams system
Mode of action	variable action on the His–Purkinje system	increase AV node refractory period	increase both AV node and His–Purkinje refractory period	increase AV node refractory period	slows AV conduction increases AV node refractory period positively inotropic
Adverse effects	quinidine—nausea, diarrhoea; procainamide—development of antinuclear antibodies and SLE; flecainide—higher incidence of proarrhythmic effects than other class I drugs; all may lengthen QT and cause torsades; all are negatively inotropic	negatively inotropic, may induce bronchospasm, exacerbation of peripheral vascular disease	amiodarone—pulmonary fibrosis, hypo/hyperthyroidism, hepatic toxicity, cutaneous photosensitivity; corneal microdeposits (reversible), peripheral neuropathy; sotalol—as for other β-blockers; both may lengthen QT and cause torsades	verapamil and diltiazem—complete AV block, negatively inotropic	nausea, vomiting if blood levels too high, visual disturbances (xanthopsia), complete heart block

Main features of common antiarrhythmic drugs

Fig. 16.7 Main features of common antiarrhythmic drugs classed using Vaughan Williams classification. (AV, atrioventricular; SLE, systemic lupus erythematosus.)

- Flecainide is an effective agent, but is avoided in patients who have suspected ischaemic heart disease because this is thought to increase its proarrhythmic effects.

The Vaughan Williams classification of antiarrhythmic drugs allows agents to be grouped according to their mode of action on the myocardium and also makes selection of appropriate agents for the treatment of any given arrhythmia more straightforward; however, see also the Sicilian Gambit classification.

NON-PHARMACOLOGICAL TREATMENTS OF VENTRICULAR TACHYARRHYTHMIAS

Non-pharmacological treatments are used in patients who have recurrent VT or VF because:
- If successful, complete cure is achieved without the need for drugs.

- Localization of the arrhythmogenic focus is becoming possible in more cases due to increased understanding of the mechanisms of these arrhythmias.

The two methods commonly used are:
- Radiofreqency ablation.
- Implantable cardioverter defibrillator (ICD).

Radiofreqency ablation
This involves localization of the proarrhythmic focus using intracardiac electrodes introduced via a central vein followed by the use of radiofrequency energy to cauterize the myocardium in that area. The successful result is the ablation of the focus, therefore rendering the patient cured and no longer needing antiarrhythmic agents. This technique is commonly used in patients who have Wolff–Parkinson–White syndrome (a supraventricular arrhythmia) who are young and have a discreet accessory pathway that can be localized easily. Ventricular arrhythmias can also sometimes be ablated.

Implantable cardioverter defibrillators

Implantable cardioverter defibrillators (ICDs) are now being increasingly used in the treatment of sustained or life-threatening ventricular arrhythmias because they have been shown in some studies to prolong survival in such patients. These devices are slightly larger than a permanent pacemaker and are implanted in the same way (i.e. the box is situated under the pectoralis major muscle on the patient's non-dominant side and the leads are positioned in the atrium and ventricle). The device can sense VT and VF and can attempt to cardiovert the arrhythmia by pacing the ventricle or by delivering a DC shock.

The implantation and subsequent programming and monitoring of these devices should be performed in specialist centres. In addition the patients often need counselling and advice because the sensation when the ICD discharges a shock can be extremely unpleasant and comes without warning. This results in marked psychological problems in some patients.

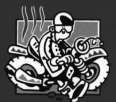

17. Cardiac Arrest and Resuscitation

Cardiopulmonary arrest results in a rapid decline in oxygen delivery to the brain. Permanent disability or death results if the period of cerebral hypoxia lasts longer than 3 minutes.

Cardiopulmonary resuscitation (CPR) is the term used to describe the maintenance of adequate breathing and circulation in a patient who cannot do so for himself.

The aim of CPR is to restore respiration and adequate cardiac output as soon as possible to prevent death or permanent disability. Cardiopulmonary resuscitation involves two types of protocol:

- Basic life support (BLS)—no special equipment required.
- Advanced life support (ALS)—requires specialist skill and equipment.

In any type of resuscitation protocol the following three areas must be assessed and supported in order of priority:

- Airway.
- Breathing.
- Circulation.

BASIC LIFE SUPPORT

Basic life support refers to the maintenance and support of airway, breathing, and circulation without the aid of any specialized equipment. The aim of BLS is to maintain adequate ventilation and cardiac output until the underlying cause can be reversed.

There are a number of points to note relating to Fig. 17.1:

- If trauma to the cervical spine is a possibility the airway should be maintained without tilting the head.
- If there are two operators one should go for help as soon as possible. If there is only one it is generally agreed now that the victim can be left and the operator should go for help once it has been established that the victim is not breathing. If, however, the victim is a child, or collapse was due to trauma or drowning, then 1 min of CPR should be given before the operator goes for help—in these situations the collapse is likely to be due to

respiratory arrest and the rescue breaths if given early will improve prognosis.

- Each rescue breath, is given by mouth to mouth inflation with the nose occluded, and should deliver approximately 500 ml expired air into the lungs of the victim. The operator should watch the chest wall of the victim to ensure that it rises and falls with each breath. Each breath will take approximately 1–1.5 s. It is important to allow the chest wall to fall back completely before taking the next breath.
- Assessment of the carotid pulse should take no more than 10 s.
- If there is no pulse, chest compressions are performed by placing the heel of the hand over the lower half of the sternum two fingerbreadths above the xiphoid process. Enough pressure should be applied to depress the sternum 4–5 cm and no more. The operator should be vertically above the victim's chest and the arms should be kept straight. The rate of compressions should be 100/min. After each compression the pressure should be released and the chest wall allowed to rise back up.

Principal of chest compressions

The current theory suggests that chest compression increases intrathoracic pressure and it is this that propels blood out of the thorax. The veins collapse whereas the arteries remain patent therefore flow is in a forward direction.

The function and features of the recovery position are shown in Fig. 17.2.

The final examinations are likely to test BLS techniques so practice these until you are competent. Inability to perform BLS satisfactorily in finals almost always results in a fail.

Management of upper airway obstruction by foreign material

The management of choking in a conscious victim although not strictly BLS is extremely important because it is a common occurrence both in the community and in the hospital where aspiration of stomach contents or blood may occur (Fig. 17.3).

Points to note in the management of choking:
- If the patient becomes cyanosed then immediate positive action is needed with administration of oxygen and back blows followed by the Heimlich manoeuvre.

- Back blows are performed during expiration either with the patient standing or sitting and with the head bent down below the level of the chest.
- Heimlich manoeuvre—this may be performed with the patient standing, sitting, or lying down.

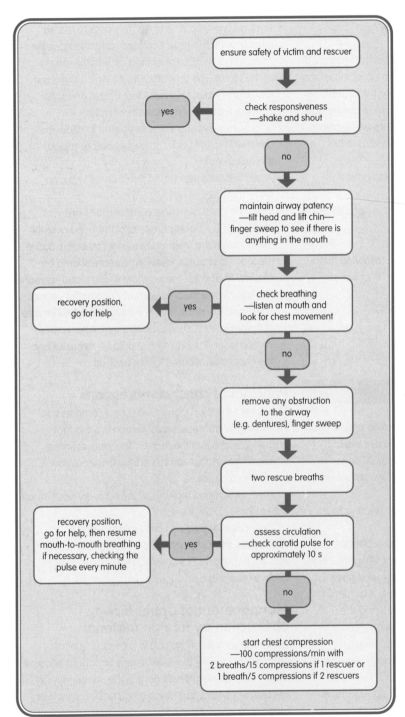

Fig. 17.1 Algorithm for adult basic life support.

ensure safety of victim and rescuer

check responsiveness
—shake and shout

yes

no

maintain airway patency
—tilt head and lift chin—
finger sweep to see if there is
anything in the mouth

check breathing
—listen at mouth and
look for chest movement

recovery position,
go for help

yes

no

remove any obstruction
to the airway
(e.g. dentures), finger sweep

two rescue breaths

assess circulation
—check carotid pulse for
approximately 10 s

recovery position,
go for help, then resume
mouth-to-mouth breathing
if necessary, checking the
pulse every minute

yes

no

start chest compression
—100 compressions/min with
2 breaths/15 compressions if 1 rescuer or
1 breath/5 compressions if 2 rescuers

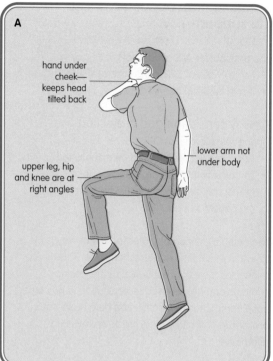

Sharp upward pressure is applied in the midline just beneath the diaphragm with the operator behind the patient. This procedure may result in damage to abdominal viscera and should not be attempted in small children or pregnant women.

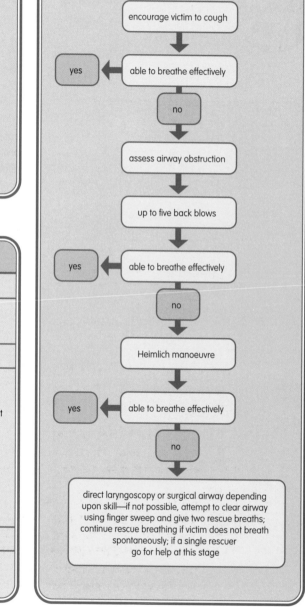

B	Function and features of the recovery position

Function

keeps airway straight
allows tongue to fall forward and not obstruct airway
minimizes risk of aspiration of gastric contents

Main features

remove victim's spectacles
ensure airway is open by lifting chin
kneel beside victim
tuck one hand under the victim's buttock (arm should be straight with palm facing up)
bring other forearm across patient's chest and hold back of hand against the victim's nearest cheek
with your other hand bring far leg into a bent position with foot still on the ground and keeping the hand pressed against the cheek pull on the leg to roll the victim towards you onto his or her side
the upper leg should be adjusted so both the hip and the knee are at right angles

Special notes

the patient should not be lying on his or her lower arm
the hand under the cheek keeps the head tilted back so the airway remains open

Fig. 17.2 **(A)** The recovery position viewed from above.
(B) Function and features of the recovery position.

Fig. 17.3 Algorithm for the management of choking.

ADVANCED LIFE SUPPORT

The ALS method of resuscitation requires specialist training and equipment and has recently been reviewed and modified. The 1997 Resuscitation Council (UK) guidelines use a universal algorithm that is dependent upon the presence or absence of VT or VF (Fig. 17.4).

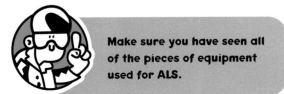

Make sure you have seen all of the pieces of equipment used for ALS.

Points to note about advanced life support
Protocol
The protocol for ALS consists of:
- 1-min cycles of CPR in the case of VT/VF.
- 3-min cycles in non-VT/VF.

Airway ventilation and protection
During these cycles of CPR:
- Adequate ventilation must be established.
- The airway must be protected by an operator (preferably an anaesthetist) who remains at the patient's head.

The optimal method of protecting the airway is by insertion of a cuffed endotracheal tube. This device minimizes the risk of aspiration of the gastric contents and allows effective ventilation to be carried out. Endotracheal intubation can be a hazardous procedure and a laryngeal mask airway is an alternative.

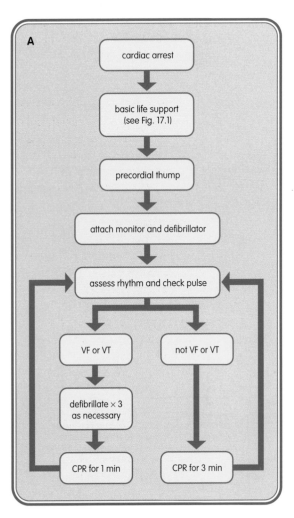

A

cardiac arrest

↓

basic life support
(see Fig. 17.1)

↓

precordial thump

↓

attach monitor and defibrillator

↓

assess rhythm and check pulse

VF or VT   not VF or VT

↓   ↓

defibrillate × 3
as necessary

↓   ↓

CPR for 1 min   CPR for 3 min

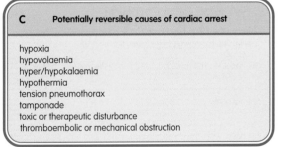

B	**Management aspects to consider during CPR**

correct reversible causes
check electrode and paddle positions and contact
check airway and oxygen
ensure there is intravenous access
apply DC shock if patient in VF
if the patient remains in shock give adrenaline every 3 min
consider giving antiarrhythmics, atropine
consider pacing
consider buffers

C	**Potentially reversible causes of cardiac arrest**

hypoxia
hypovolaemia
hyper/hypokalaemia
hypothermia
tension pneumothorax
tamponade
toxic or therapeutic disturbance
thromboembolic or mechanical obstruction

Fig. 17.4 (A) Algorithm for advanced life support. **(B)** Management aspects to consider during cardiopulmonary resuscitation (CPR). **(C)** Potentially reversible causes of cardiac arrest. (VF, ventricular fibrillation; VT, ventricular tachycardia.)

> **Regardless of the setting it is crucial that BLS is commenced immediately and once a cardiac monitor is available, that defibrillation of VT/VF is administered immediately. It is these two factors that affect the eventual outcome of resuscitation.**

Intravenous access must also be established either via a large peripheral vein or preferably via a central vein.

Placement of defibrillator paddles

Placement of the defibrillator paddles is important because only a small proportion of the energy reaches the myocardium during transthoracic defibrillation and every effort should be made to maximize this:

- The right paddle should be placed below the clavicle in the midclavicular line.
- The left paddle should be placed on the lower rib cage on the anterior axillary line.

The VT/VF arm of the ALS algorithm

The three initial shocks are usually 200, 200, and 360 J. Subsequent shocks are usually all 360 J. After each shock the monitor should be watched:

- If the rhythm remains VF/VT then the CPR and defibrillation sequence should be followed for four cycles.
- If the arrhythmia persists at this stage antiarrhythmics can be used. Intravenous lignocaine, amiodarone, or bretylium can be used as can other agents. (No one agent has been found to be better in this situation.)
- If the monitor shows a flat line after defibrillation this does not necessarily mean asystole has occurred. It is not uncommon for a period of myocardial stunning to occur after defibrillation and the screen should be watched for one full sweep.

- If the flat line persists, CPR should be carried out for 1 min before adrenaline is given to allow the period of stunning to pass.

The non-VT/VF arm of the ALS algorithm

This arm includes asystole, electromechanical dissociation, and profound bradyarrhythmias. Prognosis for patients in this arm is much poorer than in the VF/VT arm. Defibrillation is not required unless VT/VF supervenes and 3-min cycles of CPR are given. During the 3 min possible underlying causes must be excluded or treated:

- Asystole is treated initially with intravenous atropine at a maximum total dose of 3 mg and intravenous adrenaline 1 mg. During subsequent cycles of CPR adrenaline may be repeated, but not the atropine.
- Bradyarrhythmias are treated initially with atropine in the same way. Patients who have bradyarrhythmia may benefit from insertion of a temporary pacing wire.

Electromechanical dissociation (EMD) occurs when there is a regular rhythm on the monitor (that is not VT), but no cardiac output arising from it. Underlying causes must be sought because these may be easily treated. The following are possible underlying causes of EMD:

- Hypovolaemia—rapid administration of intravenous fluids required.
- Electrolyte imbalance (e.g. hypokalaemia, hypocalcaemia).
- Tension pneumothorax—suspect in trauma cases or after insertion of central line; also seen spontaneously in fit young men. Look for absence of chest movements and breath sounds on one side. Treat with cannula into the pleural space at the second intercostal space in mid-clavicular line followed by insertion of chest drain.
- Cardiac tamponade—suspect in trauma cases and post-thoracotomy patients. Need rapid insertion of pericardial drain.
- Pulmonary embolism—if strongly suspected thrombolysis should be administered.

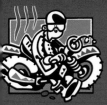

18. Bradyarrhythmias

DEFINITION OF BRADYARRHYTHMIAS

The bradyarrhythmias (Fig. 18.1) are slow rhythms.

SINUS BRADYCARDIA

Sinus bradycardia occurs when the resting heart rate is less than 60 beats/min when the patient is awake. In most cases it is asymptomatic and of no consequence (Fig. 18.2).

In pathological situations and rarely in sinus bradycardia with no obvious cause symptoms may occur. These may take the form of:

- Syncope (Stokes–Adams attacks).
- Hypotension.
- Dyspnoea due to cardiac failure.

In these circumstances treatment of the bradycardia with intravenous atropine or insertion of a temporary pacing wire may be indicated to speed the heart rate until the underlying condition is treated.

The pacing wire may be ventricular or atrial because the atrioventricular node is conducting impulses normally.

SINUS NODE DISEASE

The sinoatrial (SA) node is the natural cardiac pacemaker. It is a crescent shaped structure and is approximately 1 mm by 3 mm in size.

The location of the SA node is at the junction of the right atrium and the superior vena cava just below the epicardial surface.

Impulses are generated at the sinus node the rate of these is determined by both vagal and sympathetic tone. The impulses are then conducted via the atrial myocardium to the atrioventricular (AV) node.

Bradyarrhythmias	
Bradyarrhythmia	Features
sinus bradycardia	heart rate <60 beats/min during the day
sinoatrial node disease and sick sinus syndrome	prolonged PP interval, may be associated with tachyarrhythmias intermittently tachy–brady syndrome
first degree heart block	PR interval >0.20 s
second degree heart block —Mobitz type I	Wenckebach phenomenon— progressive prolongation of PR interval with eventual dropped beat
second degree heart block —Mobitz type II	dropped beats, no prolongation of PR interval
second degree heart block —2:1 heart block/ 3:1 heart block	every second or third beat conducted, the rest are not
complete heart block, third degree heart block	complete AV dissociation
asystole	no beats conducted, no ventricular activity

Fig. 18.1 Bradyarrhythmias listed in ascending order of electrical dysfunction. (AV, atrioventricular.)

Causes of sinus bradycardia
Physiological
atheletes young adults during sleep (rate can drop to 35–40 beats/min)
Pathological
hypothermia raised intracranial pressure hypothyroidism cholestatic jaundice ischaemic heart disease affecting the SA node (in 60% of patients the SA node is supplied by right coronary artery) drugs (e.g. β-blockers, antiarrhythmic agents) in the elderly—due to fibrosis of SA node

Fig. 18.2 Causes of sinus bradycardia. (SA, sinoatrial.)

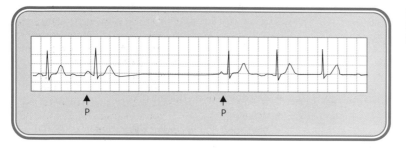

Fig. 18.3 Sinus pause or arrest. Note the interval of more than 2 s between P waves.

Disease of the SA node may be due to:
- Ischaemia and infarction.
- Degeneration and fibrosis.
- Excessive vagal stimulation.
- Myocarditis.

This may result in pauses between consecutive P waves (>2 s). There are different degrees of SA node conduction abnormality:

- Sinoatrial exit block—there is an absence of the expected P wave but the following one occurs at the expected time (i.e. the pauses are exact multiples of the basic PP interval.)
- Sinus pause or sinus arrest (Fig. 18.3)—this occurs when the interval between the P waves is longer than 2 s and is not a multiple of the basic PP interval.

Tachybrady syndrome (sick sinus syndrome)

This is a combination of sinus node disease and abnormal tachyarrhythmias. Ischaemia is a common cause for this syndrome, which occurs in the elderly.

Management

Patients who have symptomatic sinus pauses or evidence of recurrent sinus pauses require permanent pacing with either an atrial pacemaker (if there is no evidence of AV node disease) or a dual chamber pacemaker. Ventricular pacemakers are usually reserved only for very frail and elderly patients or those who have atrial fibrillation because they do not improve prognosis and are associated with fatigue and lethargy (i.e. the pacemaker syndrome, which may result from the loss of the atrial component of cardiac output).

Antiarrhythmic drugs may also be needed if the patient has sick sinus syndrome. It is important to insert a pacemaker before commencing these because they will make the SA node conduction defect worse.

ATRIOVENTRICULAR BLOCK

The AV node is a complex structure that lies in the right atrial wall on the septal surface between the ostium of the coronary sinus and the septal leaflet of the tricuspid valve; in 90% of patients the AV node is supplied by the right coronary artery. The rest are supplied via the circumflex coronary artery.

The AV node acts as a physiological gearbox conducting impulses from the atria to the ventricular conductive tissue.

First degree atrioventricular block

In this conduction disturbance (Fig. 18.4) conduction time through the AV node is prolonged, but all impulses are conducted. The PR interval is longer than 0.22 s.

This condition does not require treatment in a healthy patient but should be watched because it may herald greater degrees of block (this occurs in approximately 40% of cases)

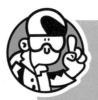

In a patient who has infective endocarditis serial ECGs are performed to observe the PR interval. Prolongation of this can occur secondary to formation of a paravalvular abscess and this usually heralds rapid development of complete heart block and valve dehiscence. In these patients progressive prolongation of the PR interval therefore requires an urgent echocardiogram and temporary pacing wire.

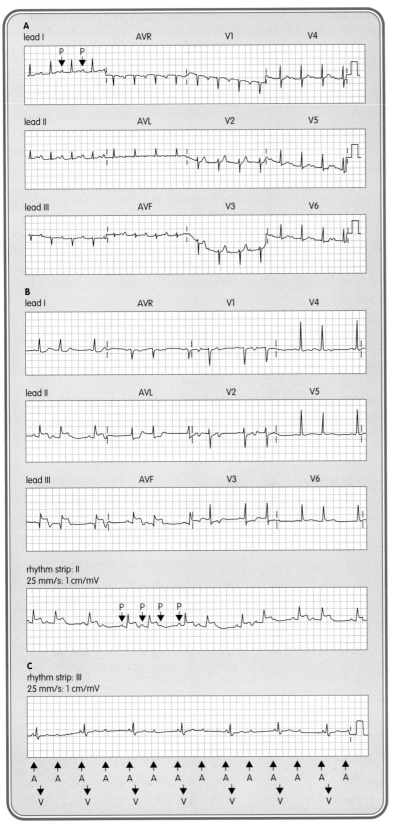

Fig. 18.4 ECGS of bradyarrhythmias. **(A)** First degree heart block. Note the long PR interval. **(B)** Mobitz type 1 (Wenckebach) partial heart block caused by inferior myocardial infarction (raised ST segments in leads II, III, and AVF). **(C)** 2:1 heart block; arrows point to dropped P waves. There are two P waves (A) from the atrium for every QRS (V) from the ventricles.

Second degree atrioventricular block
In this type of block some impulses are not conducted from the atria to the ventricles.

Mobitz type 1 heart block —Wenckebach phenomenon
Wenckebach phenomenon is characterized by progressive prolongation of the PR interval, eventually resulting in a dropped P wave. The cycle is then repeated.

This is a common phenomenon and can occur in any cardiac tissue including the SA node.

Wenckebach phenomenon can occur in atheletes and children and is due to high vagal tone. It is usually benign and is not usually an indication for pacing.

When it occurs following an inferior myocardial infarction pacing is not usually required unless it is symptomatic. In anterior myocardial infarction any newly developed heart block suggests massive septal necrosis and temporary pacing is required.

Mobitz type 2 heart block
The PR interval remains constant and P waves are dropped intermittently.

This type of heart block carries a risk of progressing to complete heart block and requires insertion of a pacemaker.

2:1 or 3:1 heart block
This represents a more advanced degree of block and requires pacing because there is a high risk of complete heart block.

Third degree or complete heart block
Complete heart block (Fig. 18.5) results in dissociation of the atria from the ventricles.

The ECG shows the P waves and the QRS waves are independent from each other. The P and QRS complexes are regular, but bear no temporal relationship to one another.

On examination there may be classical features:
- The first heart sound has a variable intensity.
- There are intermittent cannon waves in the jugular venous pulse. These correspond to a large a wave caused by the right atrial contraction against a closed tricuspid valve.

Management depends upon the underlying cause:
- After an inferior myocardial infarction a temporary pacemaker should be inserted. A significant proportion of these cases revert back to normal conduction within a few weeks and a permanent pacemaker is often not needed. If the heart block is due to drugs (e.g. β-blockers) it may resolve once these are withdrawn.
- After an anterior myocardial infarction or in any other situation a permanent pacemaker will be required and should be inserted immediately (unless the patient is unstable in which case a temporary wire is inserted first followed by a permanent system some days later).

Bradyarrhythmias do not usually compromise cardiac output if the rate is over 50/min and the ventricles have normal function.

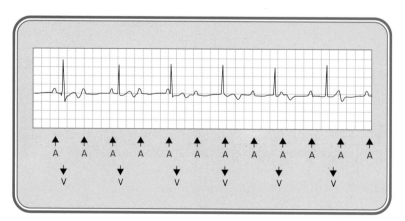

Fig. 18.5 Complete heart block. Atrial P waves (A) and ventricular QRS (V) complexes are completely dissociated.

BUNDLE BRANCH BLOCK

Bundle branch block is an interventricular conduction disturbance. The bundle of His arises from the AV node and at the level of the the top of the muscular interventricular septum it divides into left and right bundle branches (Fig. 18.6), which supply the left and right ventricles respectively. The left bundle divides again into anterior and posterior divisions.

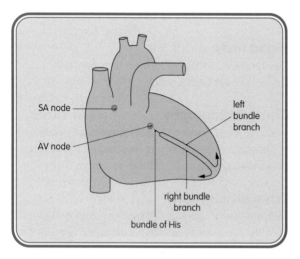

Fig. 18.6 Location of conductive tissue in the heart. (AV node, atrioventricular node; SA node, sinoatrial node.)

Damage to one or more of these bundles due to ischaemia or infarction (or any other condition disturbing electrical conduction; see SA node disease earlier in this chapter) results in a characteristic ECG picture as the pattern of depolarization of the ventricles is altered.

In either complete left or complete right bundle branch block the QRS complex is widened to greater than 0.12 s.

Left bundle branch block

In the normal situation the septum is depolarized from left to right. If the left bundle is blocked the septum is depolarized from right to left and the right ventricle depolarized before the left. This results in the classical M-shaped complex in lead V6 (Fig. 18.7).

Remember that V6 is on the left side of the chest and that a positive deflection occurs when current flows towards the lead. The initial upstroke is due to septal depolarization from right to left and therefore towards lead V6. Depolarization of the right ventricle occurs next which is in a centre to right direction and therefore causes a negative deflection. Finally the left ventricle is depolarized, which is from right to left, causing the final upstroke.

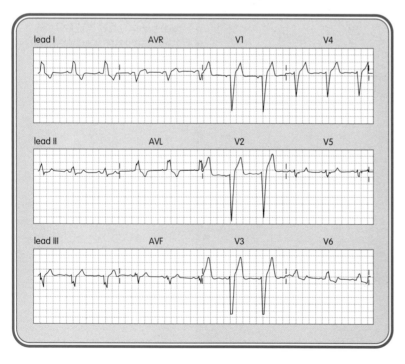

Fig. 18.7 Complete left bundle branch block. This is characterized by widening of the QRS complex. The second half in time of the QRS is positive in I (to the left) and negative in V1 (posterior) (i.e. the delayed depolarization is to the left ventricle). Note the widened complexes and the M-shaped complexes in V6.

It is possible to see isolated block of the left anterior or left posterior fascicles of the left bundle branch on the ECG. Left anterior hemiblock causes a left axis deviation on the ECG and left posterior hemiblock causes right axis deviation.

Right bundle branch block

This results in the classical RSR pattern in lead V1 and V2 (Fig. 18.8), which lies to the right of the left ventricle. The septum is depolarized from left to right as normal (resulting in an upstroke in V1), but as there is no conduction down the right bundle the left ventricle depolarizes first, which causes a current to the left resulting in a negative stroke in V1. Finally the delayed right ventricular depolarization of the right ventricle occurs causing another upstroke in V1.

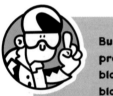

Bundle branch block may progress to complete heart block; intermittent heart block should be suspected in patients who present with syncope and bundle branch block.

INVESTIGATION OF BRADYARRHYTHMIAS

Electrocardiography

This may show evidence of heart block. However, if the heart block is intermittent the ECG may be normal.

In a patient who has unexplained syncope it is important to exclude intermittent conduction disturbances using continuous ambulatory ECG monitoring. These devices can be used to record the ECG over at least 24 hours continuously.

Blood tests

Liver function and thyroid function tests may reveal causes of sinus bradycardia.

Chest radiography

This may reveal cardiomegaly in patients who have ischaemic cardiomyopathy or myocarditis. Pulmonary oedema may be a result of the bradycardia.

Echocardiography

This may reveal regional wall hypokinesia due to areas of ischaemia or infarction. This is especially relevant if it involves the septum.

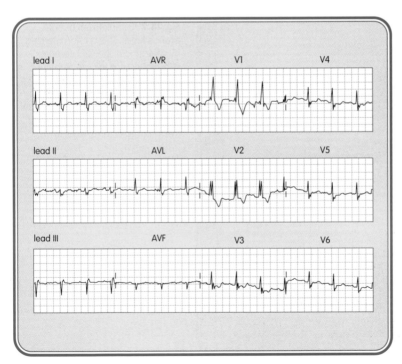

Fig. 18.8 Right bundle branch block. Note the wide QRS. The late part of the QRS in time is negative in I (i.e. to the right) and positive in V1 (i.e. anterior). The delayed depolarization is to the right ventricle. Note the widened QRS complexes and the RSR pattern in V1 and V2.

Electrophysiological studies

These studies involve inserting multiple electrodes into the heart via the great veins and positioning them at various intracardiac sites. Electrical activity can then be recorded from the atria, ventricles, bundle of His, etc. to provide information on the type of conduction defect or rhythm disturbance.

These studies are used mostly to:
- Elucidate the mechanism of tachyarrhythmias.
- Therapeutically to terminate a tachyarrhythmia by overdrive pacing or shock.
- Therapeutically to ablate an area of myocardium thought to be propagating a recurrent tachyarrhythmia.
- Diagnostically to evaluate the risk of sudden cardiac death in patients who have possible ventricular tachyarrhythmias.
- Diagnostically to determine conduction defects in patients who have recurrent syncope.

PACEMAKERS

Indications for a permanent pacemaker

A pacemaker is used to deliver electric stimuli via leads in contact with the heart. The leads not only deliver energy, but are also able to sense spontaneous electrical activity from the heart. The aim of inserting a pacemaker is to mimic as closely as possible the normal electrical activity of the heart in a patient who has a potentially life-threatening conduction disturbance. The indications for a permanent pacemaker are listed in Fig. 18.9.

Indications for temporary pacing

The following indications for temporary pacing are appropriate:
- All of the above (see Fig. 18.9) if there is no facility for permanent pacing immediately available.
- Drug-induced symptomatic bradyarrhythmias— a temporary wire is used until the effect of the drug has worn off, for example after a trial or overdose of a β-blocker (β-adrenoceptor antagonist).
- Heart block after inferior myocardial infarction.

Pacemaker insertion

Both temporary and permanent pacemakers are inserted via a venous route by introducing first a sheath and then a pacing wire into one of the great veins.

Permanent pacemakers are most often inserted into the cephalic, subclavian, or internal jugular veins. In an emergency situation a temporary wire may be inserted into the internal jugular, subclavian, or femoral vein.

In the case of the temporary pacemaker the pacemaker box sits externally. In the case of the permanent pacemaker it is buried under the fat

Indications for a permanent pacemaker
complete AV block—should be permanently paced whether symptomatic or not
Mobitz type 2 block and 2:1 and 3:1 block
symptomatic bifascicular BBB (i.e. RBBB and left anterior or posterior hemiblock)
trifascicular block, whether symptomatic or not (i.e. first degree heart block, RBBB, and left anterior or posterior hemiblock, or first degree block and LBBB)
sinus node pauses +/– tachycardia
symptomatic sinus bradycardia with no treatable cause
after inferior MI with persistent complete heart block or persistent Mobitz type 2 block after trial with temporary pacing wire for at least 2 weeks
after anterior MI with persistent complete heart block or persistent Mobitz type 2 block: trial with temporary pacing is unnecessary as conduction very rarely recovers
symptomatic bradyarrhythmia following drug treatment of a serious tachyarrhythmia: continue the antiarrhythmic drug and combine with a permanent pacemaker

Fig. 18.9 Indications for a permanent pacemaker. (LBBB, left bundle branch block; MI, myocardial infarction; RBBB, right bundle branch block.)

and subcutaneous tissue overlying one of the pectoralis major muscles (usually on the patient's non-dominant side).

Complications of pacemaker insertion

The following are recognized complications of pacemaker insertion:

- Complications of wire insertion such as pneumothorax, haemorrhage, brachial plexus injury (during subclavian vein puncture), arrhythmias as the wire is manipulated inside the heart, and infection (may progress to infective endocarditis).
- Complications of permanent pacemaker box positioning (e.g. haematoma formation, infection and erosion of the box through the skin).
- Difficulties with the wire such as wire displacement and loss of ability to pace or sense (need to reposition wire), fracture of the wire insulation (usually due to tight sutures or friction against the clavicle—need to replace wire), and perforation of myocardium (uncommon unless after myocardial infarction when the myocardium is friable—need to reposition wire).

Types of pacemaker

Pacemakers are classified according to a four letter code (Fig. 18.10).

Ventricular pacemakers stimulate ventricular contraction only and patients who have these have no atrial contribution to the cardiac output. The atrial contribution can, however, be very important (up to 25% of total cardiac output). It is generally accepted now that a dual chamber pacemaker should be fitted in patients in whom the atrium can be paced and sensed.

Patients who have chronic atrial fibrillation cannot have an atrial wire because the constant random electrical activity cannot be appropriately sensed.

Pacemaker syndrome

Permanent single chamber right ventricular pacing in a patient who has intact atrial function can lead to atrial activation by retrograde conduction from the ventricle—so-called pacemaker syndrome. There is a cannon wave with every beat, pulmonary arterial pressure rises, and cardiac output is impaired. This is managed by replacing the pacemaker with a dual chamber device.

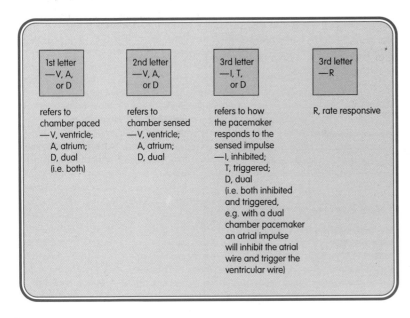

Fig. 18.10 Classification of pacemakers.

1st letter —V, A, or D	2nd letter —V, A, or D	3rd letter —I, T, or D	3rd letter —R
refers to chamber paced —V, ventricle; A, atrium; D, dual (i.e. both)	refers to chamber sensed —V, ventricle; A, atrium; D, dual	refers to how the pacemaker responds to the sensed impulse —I, inhibited; T, triggered; D, dual (i.e. both inhibited and triggered, e.g. with a dual chamber pacemaker an atrial impulse will inhibit the atrial wire and trigger the ventricular wire)	R, rate responsive

19. Cardiac Failure

DEFINITION OF CARDIAC FAILURE

Cardiac failure is the inability of the heart to adequately perfuse metabolizing tissues. The most common cause of this is myocardial failure, which can be caused by a wide variety of disease states.

Myocardial failure may affect the left and right ventricles individually or both together. Left ventricular failure (LVF) if left untreated will lead to right ventricular failure (RVF) due to high right ventricular pressure load. Very occasionally there is no abnormality of myocardial function, but cardiac failure occurs. This is due to a sudden excessive high demand on the heart—so-called high-output cardiac failure (Fig. 19.1) or acute pressure load.

For the remainder of this chapter myocardial failure will be discussed.

PATHOPHYSIOLOGY OF CARDIAC FAILURE

Normal myocardial response to work

During exercise and other stresses there is an increased adrenergic stimulation of the myocardium and cardiac pacemaker tissue. This results in tachycardia and increased myocardial contractility.

An increase in venous return causes an increased end-diastolic volume of the left ventricle resulting in stretching of the myocytes. This stretch causes an increase in myocardial performance—as predicted by the Frank–Starling law (Fig. 19.2).

Causes of high output cardiac failure
thyrotoxicosis
sepsis
chronic anaemia
Paget's disease of bone
beriberi
arteriovenous malformations
phaeochromocytoma

Fig. 19.1 Causes of high-output cardiac failure.

At the same time vasodilatation in the exercising muscles reduces peripheral vascular resistance resulting in a marked increase in cardiac output with relatively little increase in systemic blood pressure.

The terms 'preload' and 'afterload' are commonly used. Load is a force—in this case the force in the wall of the cardiac chambers.
Preload = diastolic force.
Afterload = systolic force. Preload and afterload always change together because of the LaPlace relationship (e.g. increasing venous return increases volume and therefore systolic wall force). Vasodilatation shifts blood from the heart and decreases diastolic and systolic wall force.

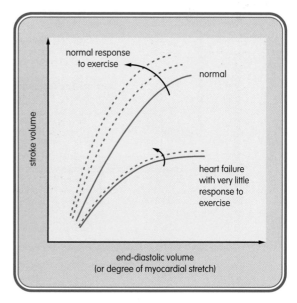

Fig. 19.2 Relationship between end-diastolic volume and stroke volume in normal and failing myocardium (Frank–Starling relationship).

The failing heart's response to work

The adrenergic system is already at an increased level of activity in cardiac failure in an attempt to boost cardiac output. During stress this stimulation increases, but cardiac reserve does not permit a significant increase in contractility. The result is tachycardia with its increased energy consumption and a small increase in cardiac output (Fig. 19.3).

Similarly the response to increased myocardial stretch is impaired in the failing heart. During stress the impairment results in inadequate contractile response and a large increase in pulmonary capillary pressure (back pressure). This predisposes to the development of pulmonary oedema.

The elevated catecholamine activity may result in peripheral vasoconstriction. Cardiac output is redistributed towards vital organs (e.g. the brain and heart) with vasoconstriction in the skin and skeletal muscle, therefore the blood flow to less crucial organs is reduced, and this underperfusion leads to formation of lactic acid and weakness and fatigue—classical symptoms in all patients who have cardiac failure.

The result is:
- An inadequate myocardial response to stress.
- Increased and wasteful myocardial energy consumption.
- Possible pulmonary oedema.

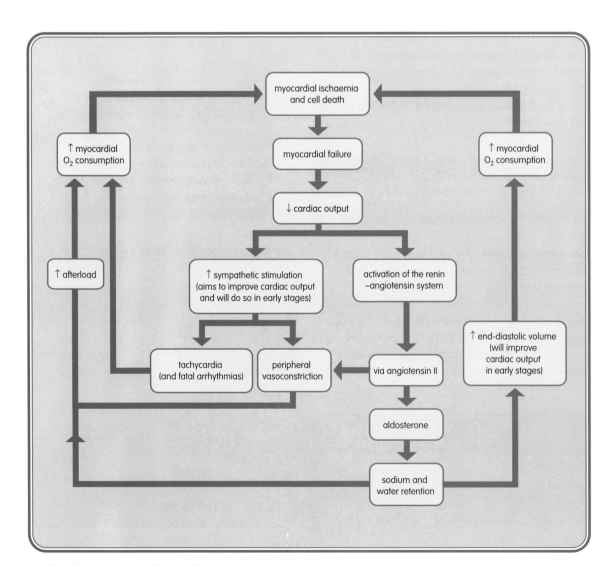

Fig. 19.3 Pathophysiology of heart failure.

Salt and water retention in cardiac failure

Salt and water retention causes the characteristic raised jugular venous pressure (JVP) and oedema of congestive cardiac failure (CCF).

The renin–angiotensin system is activated in cardiac failure for two reasons:
- Stimulation of the β_1-adrenergic receptors on the juxtaglomerular apparatus.
- Reduced renal perfusion leads to activation of the baroreceptors in the renal arterioles so stimulating renin production.

Renin acts to convert angiotensinogen to angiotensin I. The subsequent action of angiotensin-converting enzyme (predominantly in the lung) converts angiotensin I to angiotensin II.

Angiotensin II has a variety of actions:
- It is a potent vasoconstrictor.
- It may increase noradrenaline release (which in turn causes vasoconstriction and myocardial stimulation).
- It is the major stimulus for aldosterone release from the adrenal cortex. Aldosterone causes sodium retention in the distal convoluted tubule. Water is retained with the sodium resulting in increased intravascular volume, which leads to increased cardiac load, so exacerbating cardiac failure.

Other neurohumoral factors

Cardiac failure is still a relatively poorly understood field and as our understanding improves it becomes apparent that many different hormones and chemical messengers have a role to play. You will hear of these being referred to as 'neurohumoral factors'—this term is fine to use so long as you appreciate that the identity of all these factors is not known and its not known exactly how many there are.

Natriuretic peptides, cytokines, and endothelin are all thought to have a role in cardiac failure.

Natriuretic peptides
There are three such peptides known currently:
- Atrial natriuretic peptide (ANP).
- Brain natriuretic peptide (BNP).
- C-natriuretic peptide (C-NP).

Both ANP and BNP causes sodium excretion (natriuresis) resulting in water excretion and also

peripheral vasodilatation, therefore reducing cardiac load. The exact role of C-NP is unclear.

Levels of all three peptides are increased in patients who are in cardiac failure. It is generally accepted that these peptides play a protective role in cardiac failure by attempting to break the vicious cycle illustrated in Fig. 20.3.

Cytokines
Cytokines (such as tumour necrosis factor-α) are thought to be involved in causing cardiac dysfunction. Levels are increased in patients who have cardiac failure.

Other mediators, in particular growth factors, may be involved in myocardial remodelling and hypertrophy as a response to cardiac dysfunction.

Endothelin
This peptide is a powerful vasoconstrictor. It is produced by endothelial cells and there are a number of different subtypes. Endothelin levels are raised in patients who have cardiac failure. The resulting increase in load may cause increased myocardial strain in cardiac failure.

CAUSES OF CARDIAC FAILURE

Any cardiac disease can lead to cardiac failure, but a few common causes are:
- Ischaemic heart disease—remember that a right ventricular infarction will give isolated RVF which requires different acute management to LVF.
- Valve disease—aortic valve disease will lead to CCF as will MR. Remember that mitral stenosis causes RVF, but leaves the left ventricle unharmed.
- Hypertensive heart disease.
- Cardiomyopathy—secondary to viral myocarditis, drugs, inflammatory disorders, etc. (not common).

Precipitants
In most cases an acute exacerbation of cardiac failure is related to a precipitating event other than the underlying cause. Common precipitants are:
- Reduction of or non-compliance with therapy.
- Recent infection—especially pulmonary infection (which patients with cardiac failure are prone to). Infection increases metabolic rate and causes tachycardia and both increase demand on the heart.

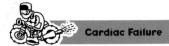

- Tachy- or bradyarrhythmias—these are common in such patients because the underlying diseases are often associated with arrhythmias. Atrial fibrillation results in a loss of the atrial component to cardiac output by reducing the efficiency of ventricular filling. Bradycardia requires an increase in stroke volume to maintain cardiac output with a lower heart rate and this may not be possible in the failing heart.

CLINICAL FEATURES OF CARDIAC FAILURE

The symptoms and signs of cardiac failure vary depending upon a number of factors:
- Severity of cardiac failure.
- Ventricles involved.
- Age of the patient.

Regardless of the cause of cardiac failure it is possible to predict the effects of cardiac failure if the mechanics of pump failure are considered. The effects can be divided into forward and backward effects.

Forward effects
Forward effects refer to the failure of the pump to provide an adequate output. This applies to the left ventricle resulting in:
- Poor renal perfusion predisposing to prerenal failure.
- Poor perfusion of extremities resulting in cold extremities.
- Increased lactic acid production in underperfused skeletal muscle leading to weakness and fatigue.
- Hypotension.

Forward failure of the right ventricle results in reduced pulmonary flow leading to dyspnoea and underfilling of the left ventricle resulting in hypotension, etc. (as above).

Backward effects
The physiological response to a failing heart is to boost output according to Starling's law due to increasing end-diastolic volume. The sodium and water retention secondary to aldosterone will serve this function. As cardiac failure worsens the pump fails to empty with each beat and this combined with progressive salt and water retention result in accumulation of blood in the atria and the venous system and therefore

tissue congestion (CCF). There is also progressive dilatation of the ventricle.

Again this applies to both left and right ventricles.

Left ventricular failure initially causes increased pulmonary venous pressure, which results in extravasation of fluid into the alveolar spaces and pulmonary oedema formation. As the pressure in the pulmonary venous system rises the backpressure affects pulmonary arterial blood and eventually the right ventricle. Undertreated LVF will therefore eventually lead to RVF.

Right ventricular failure causes increased backpressure in the venous system with resulting fluid extravasation at a number of sites:
- The peripheries—subcutaneous oedema is felt in the legs and other dependent parts.
- The liver—tender hepatomegaly is a result of hepatic congestion and may lead to cirrhotic changes.
- The abdominal cavity resulting in ascites.

Although dividing cardiac failure into right and left ventricular failure seems complicated it is worth taking the time to learn this because it makes it much easier to logically work out the cause of a given set of signs and symptoms.

Symptoms
Dyspnoea (shortness of breath), fatigue and weakness, nocturia, cough, epigastric discomfort, and anorexia are common in cardiac failure.

Dyspnoea results from pulmonary oedema, lactic acidosis, depressed respiratory muscle function, and reduced lung function. It may present in a number of ways:
- Exertional dyspnoea—as cardiac failure worsens the level of exertion required to cause dyspnoea decreases until the patient is breathless at minimal exertion (e.g. when dressing or even when speaking).
- Orthopnoea—the increased venous return when the patient lies flat is often too much for the failing heart to pump resulting in the development of pulmonary oedema. Patients who have severe LVF often sleep using several pillows to prop them up.

- Paroxysmal nocturnal dyspnoea—after being asleep for some time the patient is awakened by severe breathlessness, which is only relieved after standing or sitting upright. It is thought that this is due to pulmonary oedema due to gradual resorption of interstitial fluid overnight and nocturnal depression of respiratory function.

Fatigue and weakness result from reduced perfusion of skeletal muscles, and nocturia is due to the increased renal perfusion in the recumbent position.

Cough may be:
- A nocturnal dry cough due to bronchial oedema or cardiac asthma (bronchospasm secondary to oedema).
- Productive of pink frothy sputum due to pulmonary oedema.

> **Cough is often overlooked as a symptom of cardiac failure with the patient being investigated for a respiratory cause instead. Remember to always include cardiac failure in the differential diagnosis of cough.**

Epigastric discomfort occurs in cases of hepatic congestion. Anorexia (which may be caused by oedema of the gut), ankle swelling (due to peripheral oedema), and shortness of breath (due to inadequate pulmonary perfusion) may occur in a patient who has predominantly right-sided heart failure.

EXAMINATION OF PATIENTS WHO HAVE CARDIAC FAILURE

On observation the patient may be short of breath and cyanosed. Alternatively if the cardiac failure is relatively mild there may be no obvious abnormality at rest, but the dyspnoea may become apparent on exertion (e.g. when undressing before the examination).

Cardiac cachexia is a term used to describe cachexia seen in patients who have chronic cardiac failure; this is due to:

- Gut and liver congestion leading to anorexia.
- Increased metabolism due to increased work of breathing and increased cardiac oxygen consumption.

Cardiovascular system

On examination of the cardiovascular system (Fig. 19.4) note:
- Pulse—may be rapid, weak, and thready if there is considerable forward failure. Watch out for arrhythmias and pulsus alternans (alternate strong and weak beats), which is a sign of LVF.
- Blood pressure—this may be normal, low in forward failure, or high in the hypertensive patient (remember that hypertension is a common cause of cardiac failure.
- Jugular venous pressure—this is elevated in CCF and pure right-sided failure (the normal jugular venous pressure is 2–3 cm above the sternal angle).

> **If a raised JVP is non-pulsatile, consider superior vena caval obstruction. A pulsatile raised JVP with no oedema means right heart failure. A pulsatile raised JVP with oedema is usually due to congestive cardiac failure, but right heart failure is revealed if the JVP remains high after removal of the oedema with diuretics.**

- Carotid pulse—look for abnormal pulse character because it may reveal a possible aetiology for the cardiac failure (e.g. aortic stenosis or regurgitation).
- Apex beat—may be displaced downward and laterally in a patient who has an enlarged left ventricle. A diffuse apex beat is a sign of severe left ventricular dysfunction.
- Heart sounds—on auscultation there may be a third heart sound. Tachycardia combined with a third (or fourth heart sound) is referred to as a gallop rhythm.
- Murmurs—these may signify a possible cause of cardiac failure (e.g. aortic valve murmurs and mitral valve murmurs). Remember mitral regurgitation may

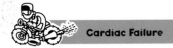
A	Consequences of left and right ventricular failure	
	LV failure	RV failure
Symptoms	dyspnoea secondary to pulmonary oedema and lactic acidosis	dyspnoea secondary to poor pulmonary perfusion
	fatigue due to poor cardiac output and lactic acidosis	fatigue due to poor LV filling (and therefore poor cardiac output and lactic acidosis)
Signs	hypotension, cold peripheries, and renal impairment—all due to poor LV output	hypotension and cold peripheries due to poor LV filling (and therefore poor LV output)
	LV 3rd heart sound—heard best at the apex	RV 3rd heart sound—very soft and best heard at the left lower sternal edge
	bilateral basal crepitations	elevated JVP
	signs of CCF—severe chronic LV failure leads to fluid retention	ascites, hepatic enlargement, and peripheral oedema

Fig. 19.4 (A) Consequences of left and right ventricular failure. One or the other will be dominant and the clinical picture varies accordingly. Often there are signs of both. **(B)** Clinical findings in a patient who has heart failure. (BP, blood pressure; CCF, congestive cardiac failure; JVP, jugular venous pressure; LV, left ventricle; RV, right ventricle.)

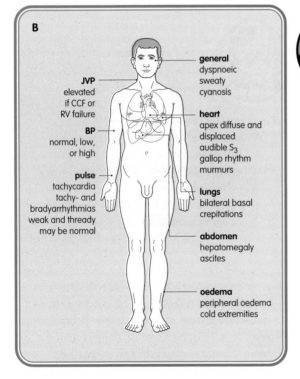

B

JVP
elevated
if CCF or
RV failure

BP
normal, low,
or high

pulse
tachycardia
tachy- and
bradyarrhythmias
weak and thready
may be normal

general
dyspnoeic
sweaty
cyanosis

heart
apex diffuse and
displaced
audible S₃
gallop rhythm
murmurs

lungs
bilateral basal
crepitations

abdomen
hepatomegaly
ascites

oedema
peripheral oedema
cold extremities

Dyspnoea secondary to pulmonary oedema is worse on lying flat and in severe cases the patient has to sit upright. In this situation it is reasonable not to ask the patient to sit at 45 degrees and to conduct the examination in the upright position.

occur as a result of left ventricular dilatation and will therefore be caused by cardiac failure and not a cause of it in some cases.

• Peripheral oedema—this may be elicited over the sacrum or over the ankle. Take care because oedema may be tender. The extent to which the oedema extends up the legs is an indication of the extent of the fluid overload.

Respiratory system

In addition to dyspnoea and possible cyanosis the patient may have bilateral basal fine end-inspiratory crepitations extending from the bases upwards. This is classical of pulmonary oedema.

In addition there may be pleural effusions and expiratory wheeze (secondary to cardiac asthma).

Gastrointestinal system

In patients who have CCF or pure RVF there may be signs of hepatomegaly and ascites.

Take care when palpating the liver or attempting to elicit the hepatojugular reflex because CCF may result in tender hepatomegaly.

INVESTIGATION OF CARDIAC FAILURE

Blood tests
Electrolytes and renal function
Hypokalaemia and hyponatraemia are common findings in patients who are on diuretic therapy. There may also be renal impairment due to hypoperfusion or diuretic therapy. Hyponatraemia may be found in patients who are not on diuretics due to sodium restriction and high circulating vasopressin levels (dilutional hyponatraemia).

Hyperkalaemia may be seen in patients who are being treated with potassium-sparing diuretics (e.g. amiloride, spironolactone) or angiotensin-converting enzyme (ACE) inhibitors (e.g. captopril, enalapril).

Full blood count
Chronic anaemia may lead to cardiac failure. There may be a leucocytosis secondary to infection, which may exacerbate cardiac failure.

Liver function tests
Liver congestion may lead to impaired hepatic funtion, resulting in elevated hepatic enzymes and bilirubin.

Arterial blood gases
These show hypoxia, hypocapnoea, and metabolic acidosis. The patient may require artificial ventilation if he or she is profoundly hypoxic.

Electrocardiography
This may be normal or may show ischaemic or hypertensive changes. Look out for evidence of arrhythmias. If these are susupected a 24-hour ECG should be performed.

Chest radiography
There may be cardiomegaly indicating a dilated left ventricle. Pulmonary oedema may be seen with prominent pulmonary veins upper lobe blood diversion and Kerley B lines (horizontal lines of fluid-filled fissures at the costophrenic angle).

Echocardiography
This is not usually an acute investigation, but it is extremely useful to evaluate the severity of LVF. The degree of left ventricular dilatation can be assessed as can the presence of pulmonary hypertension and right ventricular dilatation. Any valve lesions will be seen.

Dilatation and hypokinesis of the left ventricle is a situation predisposing to the formation of intraventricular thrombus. Transthoracic echocardiography is not a reliable method for diagnosing this, but if suspected transoesophageal echocardiography should be performed and the patient anticoagulated if intracardiac thrombus is found.

MANAGEMENT OF CARDIAC FAILURE

The most common clinical presentation seen in the outpatients department and on the ward is the patient who has chronic LVF or CCF (heart failure with fluid retention).

Before discussing this two clinical situations should be covered because they are both emergencies and make good viva questions to ask in finals.

These are
- Management of acute LVF.
- Management of acute RVF.

Management of acute left ventricular failure
This is a medical emergency that you will encounter in your first year as a house officer. You will be expected to administer all first-line treatment by yourself so it is important to know not only the drugs to use, but all the doses and routes of adminstration. This tends to be a pass/fail question in vivas.

The patient in acute LVF has pulmonary oedema and is very breathless and distressed. He or she will be hypoxic and may cough up pink frothy sputum. Forward failure may be present leading to hypotension.

Your aim is to relieve the pulmonary oedema rapidly.

If the patient has cardiogenic shock and is very hypotensive inotropic agents may be needed and you should call your registrar or senior house officer immediately because in this situation the blood pressure should be improved first.

Learn the management guide given in Fig. 19.5.

Acute left ventricular failure is a very common condition and is also a medical emergency. Rapid venodilatation is required to remove blood and fluid from the chest. It is therefore important that you know all the management steps including drugs and doses before finals.

Management of acute right ventricular failure

Patients who have an inferior or posterior myocardial infarction may present with predominantly RVF. This is not common, but it is important to recognize the signs and to know how to treat it.

Remember Starling's law of the heart where the force of contraction is proportional to the stretch applied to the muscle.

Basically it is often possible to improve function by increasing heart volume (unless the ventricle is severely dysfunctional in which case this makes no difference).

Fig. 19.5 Management of acute left ventricular failure (LVF). (CPAP, continuous positive airway pressure; IV, intravenous.)

Management of acute LVF	
Management in order	Notes
sit the patient up	to reduce venous return to the heart
administer 100% oxygen via a facial mask	improvement of arterial oxygen tension will reduce myocardial oxygen debt and improve myocardial function
establish peripheral intravenous access and administer:	
IV diamorphine 2.5–5 mg	diamorphine is a good anxiolytic and also a venodilator, so reducing load
IV metoclopramide 10 mg	metoclopramide prevents vomiting secondary to diamorphine
IV frusemide 80–100 mg	frusemide is a venodilator so its initial effect is to reduce load; it is also a powerful diuretic and will cause salt and water excretion so reducing fluid retention
	by reducing load these drugs reduce the backpressure on the pulmonary circulation and hence relieve pulmonary oedema by allowing resorption of fluid back from the extracellular to the intracellular space
insert a urinary catheter	the patient will have a diuresis and is too ill to use a bed pan; also it is important to be able to monitor fluid output to detect renal impairment early.
intravenous nitrates	given as a continuous infusion; help by vasodilating both veins and arterioles and so reducing load; the dose is titrated to prevent hypotension (a common side effect of nitrates)
CPAP	very effective—it literally pushes fluid out of the alveoli back into the circulation; specialist equipment is required
once the patient is stable continue management as for chronic left ventricular failure	

In the post-myocardial infarction patient dehydration, diuretic use, and the use of nitrates are all common. All of these conspire to reduce heart volume.

If right ventricular function is impaired a reduced heart volume has the effect of reducing function further resulting in poor left ventricular filling and hypotension. In fact an impaired right ventricle requires greater than normal filling to maintain normal output.

Treatment of acute RVF can be opposite to that of acute LVF. Fluid administration may be needed in RVF. In LVF the fluid needs to be removed.

You must be aware that hypotension after inferior myocardial infarction may be secondary to the combination of right ventricular failure and relative underfilling of the right ventricle and that the treatment of this is careful fluid challenge with central venous pressure monitoring.

Therefore a patient who has an inferior myocardial infarction and hypotension should be carefully assessed.

Provided that there is no evidence of pulmonary oedema (suggesting the presence of significant left ventricular impairment) the correct management is a gentle fluid challenge (Fig. 19.6).

Management of chronic cardiac failure
In the treatment of chronic cardiac failure:
- The main agents used are ACE inhibitors, diuretics, nitrates, and digoxin.
- Other agents used are hydralazine, β-blockers (β-adrenoceptor antagonists), and angiotensin II receptor blockers.

Angiotensin-converting enzyme inhibitors
The role of the renin–angiotensin system in cardiac failure is discussed on pp. 142–143. It is not difficult to see that inhibition of formation of angiotensin II could be beneficial by reducing systemic vasoconstriction and the sodium and water retention caused by aldosterone.

Angiotensin II increases efferent arteriolar tone and therefore increases glomerular filtration. Because ACE inhibitors remove this ability to regulate efferent

Management of acute RVF	
Management	Notes
exclude pulmonary oedema	based on chest radiography, clinical examination, arterial oxygen levels; if present it indicates coexistent LVF and a fluid challenge is unsafe in this situation without the use of inotropic agents
assess right ventricular filling	either look at the JVP or preferably insert central venous line and measure CVP
infuse 100 ml fluid (preferably colloid) over 10 min and assess BP and CVP for improvement	
continue gentle fluid challenges up to 300 ml	CVP should rise; blood pressure should also rise; if not then diagnosis of RVF is incorrect or RV function is severely impaired—need to perform echocardiography or insert Swan–Ganz catheter to confirm diagnosis by finding a low 'wedge' pressure

Fig. 19.6 Management of acute right ventricular failure (RVF). The patient will be hypotensive and have had an inferior or posterior MI. (BP, blood pressure; CVP, central venous pressure; JVP, jugular venous pressure; wedge, pulmonary capillary pressure with a Swan–Ganz balloon inflated—it reflects left atrial and pulmonary venous pressure.)

arteriolar tone glomerular filtration rate declines and renal failure ensues in patients who have renal artery stenosis or any other condition where renal blood flow is reduced (e.g. marked hypotension).

Examples of ACE inhibitors grouped according to which part of the molecule binds the zinc moiety of ACE are:

- Captopril—has a sulphydryl group.
- Enalapril, lisinopril, ramipril—carboxyl group.
- Fosinopril—phosphinic acid.

> **A dilated heart means chronic rather than acute heart failure.**

The ACE inhibitors have been shown to reduce the mortality rate for patients who have heart failure. They are the first-line drugs for all patients who have heart failure unless there is a specific contraindication (e.g. renal artery stenosis or profound hypotension).

Clinical use of angiotensin-converting enzyme inhibitors

Angiotensin-converting enzyme inhibitors are usually started at low doses because they can cause first-dose hypertension. Patients most likely to suffer from this are:

- The elderly.
- Patients who are on high doses of diuretics.

It is appropriate to admit these patients to hospital for a few hours for monitoring while the first dose is given.

> **The vast majority of patients who have cardiac failure do not require admission to hospital when starting ACE inhibitors. The first dose can be taken at night so that the patient is in bed for the duration of the first dose effect. This makes the risk of postural hypotension occurring extremely unlikely.**

Once the dose has been established renal function and electrolytes should be checked 1 week later to ensure no deterioration has taken place in renal function. Hyperkalaemia is another complication which is due to a reduction in aldosterone activity (aldosterone causes sodium absorption in exchange for potassium in the distal convoluted tubule).

Other side effects of ACE inhibitors are:

- Cough—occurs in 5% patients on these agents. It is caused by inhibition of the metabolism of bradykinin (another function of ACE). Cough usually appears in the first few weeks of treatment. This is a side effect of all drugs in this class and treatment needs to be stopped in some cases.
- Loss of taste (or a metallic taste) may occur.
- Rashes and angioedema.

Once the drug has been introduced the dose should be increased to the recommneded dose if possible (e.g. captopril 50 mg three times a day, enalapril, 10 mg twice daily).

Nitrates

The nitrates (e.g. isosorbide mononitrate and isosorbide dinitrate) are veno- and arteriolar dilators and therefore act by reducing load. Intravenous nitrates are useful in the treatment of the acutely sick patient with cardiac failure. Oral nitrates may provide some symptomatic relief in chronic cardiac failure. The combination of nitrates and hydralazine have been shown to reduce the mortality rate of cardiac failure.

Diuretics

Diuretics (Fig. 19.7) have no effect on the mortality rate of cardiac failure, but have an important role in salt and water excretion. They provide symptomatic relief.

Digoxin

Digoxin is a cardiac glycoside. This drug inhibits the sodium/potassium pump on the sarcolemmal and cell membranes. This adenosine triphosphate (ATP)-dependent pump has a role in transporting calcium out of the cell. Inhibition therefore prevents this resulting in increased intracellular calcium concentration which in cardiac muscle results in a positive inotropic effect.

In atrioventricular (AV) node tissue the effect of an increased calcium concentration is to prolong the refractory period and decrease AV node conduction

Site of action and side effects of different diuretics		
Examples	Site of action	Side effects
loop diuretics: frusemide, bumetanide, ethacrynic acid	thick ascending loop of Henle	ototoxicity with ethacrynic acid; hypokalaemia; exacerbation of gout
thiazide diuretics: bendrofluazide, hydrochlorthiazide, metalozone	distal convoluted tubule	hyperglycaemia, gout, elevated triglycerides/LDL, hypokalaemia, hyponatraemia
potassium-sparing diuretics: amiloride, spironolactone	collecting duct and distal convoluted tubule	hyperkalaemia—must not be used with ACE inhibitors

Fig. 19.7 Site of action and side effects of different diuretics. (ACE, angiotensin-converting enzyme inhibitor; low-density lipoprotein, LDL.)

velocity so slowing AV node conduction of the cardiac impulse—a negative chronotropic effect.

It is generally accepted that digoxin is an extremely useful drug in patients who have atrial fibrillation and cardiac failure, but there is no evidence to suggest that the use of digoxin as an antifailure agent alone is effective in reducing mortality rates.

Pharmacokinetics
Digoxin has a half-life of 24–36 hours and it takes 3–4 weeks time to reach a steady plasma level after oral loading. Intravenous loading speeds this up slightly because the time taken for absorption in the gut is bypassed. 40% of digoxin in the blood is protein bound.

Excretion is predominantly renal (10% excreted in the stools) and digoxin should not be used in renal failure. In mild renal impairment the dose is reduced

Side effects
Plasma levels of digoxin should be monitored and maintained at between 1 and 2 ng/mL. Blood is taken 8 hours after an oral dose. Digoxin toxicity is more likely in patients who:
- Have renal failure.
- Are hypokalaemic—digoxin competes with potassium for binding to the sodium/potassium ATPase.
- Are taking amiodarone or verapamil (which displace digoxin from protein binding sites), erythromycin (which prevents inactivation of digoxin by gut bacteria), and captopril (which reduces renal clearance of digoxin).

Signs of digoxin toxicity are:
- Bradycardia, AV block, sinus arrest.
- Nausea and vomiting.
- Xanthopsia (yellow discolouration of visualized objects).

Angiotensin II receptor blockers
There are two types of angiotensin II receptor AT1 and AT2. Losartan is a selective AT1 blocker and is the first of these drugs to be established for use as an antihypertensive. Trials are currently underway to investigate its value in the treatment of cardiac failure.

The spectrum of activity is the same as that of ACE inhibitors, but the main advantage is that these drugs do not prevent the breakdown of bradykinin so cough does not occur as a side effect.

Hydralazine
Hydralazine is a potent vasodilator, predominantly of arterioles; therefore it reduces load, which acts to improve cardiac function.

Side effects include flushing and a lupus-like syndrome.

β-Blockers
The negative inotropic effect of β-blockers has made their use in cardiac failure extremely rare until recently. Indeed medical students have always been reminded that cardiac failure is a contraindication to the use of β-blockers.

As always in medicine one can never say never and it seems that β-blockers are in fact an effective treament option in cardiac failure. As mentioned on pp. 141–142 there is a high circulating level of catecholamines in cardiac failure. There is also a downregulation of β receptors in response to this (perhaps the heart's way of protecting itself from the

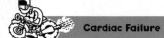

tachycardia and increased metabolic rate that results from sympathetic stimulation). Recent trials of metoprolol, bisoprolol and carvedilol have shown benefit in their use in cardiac failure and this may be for a number of reasons:

- Reduction in myocardial oxygen demand and ischaemia.
- Decreased incidence of arrhythmias.
- Peripheral vasodilatation with non-selective β-blockers that have some α blockade as well.
- Antioxidant effects (carvedilol).

Carvedilol, a non-selective β-blocker with α-blocking activity, has been shown to reduce mortality rates in chronic heart failure by over 30%.

β-Blockers must be introduced with care to patients who have heart failure because they may cause the patient's symptoms to deteriorate. There is still no evidence to suggest that they have efficacy in patients who have severe heart failure (i.e. dyspnoea at rest) or acute heart failure.

Patients who have heart failure should be stabilized with other drugs before prescribing β-blockers.

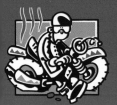

20. Cardiomyopathy

DEFINITION OF CARDIOMYOPATHY

Cardiomyopathy is heart muscle disease, often of unknown cause.

There are three types of cardiomyopathy (Fig. 20.1):
- Dilated cardiomyopathy.
- Hypertrophic obstructive cardiomyopathy (HOCM).
- Restrictive cardiomyopathy.

DILATED CARDIOMYOPATHY

The heart is dilated and has impaired function. The coronary arteries are normal.

Probable causes of dilated cardiomyopathy include:
- Alcohol.
- Viral infection (echovirus, coxsackievirus, and enteroviruses most likely).
- Untreated hypertension.
- Autoimmune disease.
- Thyrotoxicosis
- Drugs (cocaine, adriamycin, cyclophosphamide, lead).
- Haemachromatosis.
- Acquired immunodeficiency syndrome (AIDS).

Clinical features

Progressive biventricular cardiac failure leads to:
- Fatigue.
- Dyspnoea.

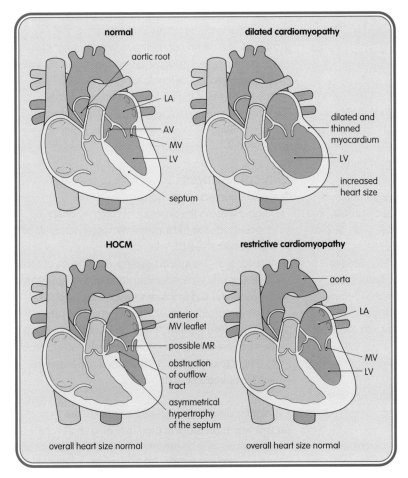

Fig. 20.1 Different types of cardiomyopathy. (AV, aortic valve; HOCM, hypertrophic obstructive cardiomyopathy; LA, left atrium; LV, left ventricle; MR, mitral regurgitation; MV, mitral valve.)

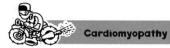

- Peripheral oedema.
- Ascites.

Other complications secondary to the progressive dilatation of the ventricles include:
- Mural thrombi with systemic or pulmonary embolization.
- Dilatation of the tricuspid and mitral valve rings leading to functional valve regurgitation.
- Atrial fibrillation.
- Ventricular tachyarrhythmias and sudden death.

Investigation
Investigations to aid diagnosis are listed below.

Chest radiography
This may show:
- Enlarged cardiac shadow.
- Signs of pulmonary oedema (upper lobe blood diversion, interstitial shadowing at the bases).
- Pleural effusions.

Electrocardiography
Electrocardiography may highlight:
- Tachycardia.
- Poor R wave progression across the chest leads.

Echocardiography
Points to consider with echocardiography include can the dilated ventricles be easily visualized? and can the regurgitant valves be seen?

Occasionally intracardiac thrombus may be seen (transthoracic echocardiography is not a reliable method for diagnosing this, but it can be accurately diagnosed by transoesophageal echocardiography.

Cardiac catheterization
This is important to exclude coronary artery disease (the most common cause of ventricular dysfunction).

Endomyocardial biopsy may be carried out during this procedure and may occasionally provide clues to a diagnosis (e.g. a viral RNA or evidence of iron overload in haemachromatosis).

Blood tests
Viral titres may be useful and also thyroid function tests.

Management
The management plan follows four basic steps (the same applies for any other case of cardiac failure):

- Search for and treat any underlying cause (e.g. stop alcohol).
- Treat cardiac failure (diuretics, angiotensin-converting enzyme inhibitors, nitrates).
- Treat any arrhythmias (digoxin or amiodarone for atrial fibrillation, amiodarone for ventricular arrhythmias).
- Anticoagulate with warfarin to prevent mural thrombi.

If the cardiac failure does not respond to the above steps and the patient is a suitable candidate then cardiac transplantation may be a possible option.

HYPERTROPHIC OBSTRUCTIVE CARDIOMYOPATHY

This disorder is characterized by asymmetrical hypertrophy of the cardiac septum—the cardiac septum is hypertrophied compared to the free wall of the left ventricle.

Hypertrophic obstructive cardiomyopathy is inherited as an autosomally dominant trait with equal sex incidence. The genetic abnormality is the subject of much current research and it seems that different genes may be involved in different families.

The myocytes of the left ventricle are abnormally thick when examined microscopically. This makes left ventricular filling more difficult than normal and grossly disordered.

Clinical features
There are four main symptoms:
- Angina (even in the absence of coronary artery disease)—due to the increased oxygen demands of the hypertrophied muscle.
- Palpitations—there is an increased incidence of atrial fibrillation and ventricular arrhythmias in this condition.
- Syncope and sudden death, which may be due to left ventricular outflow tract obstruction by the hypertrophied septum or to a ventricular arrhythmia.
- Dyspnoea—due to the stiff left ventricle, which leads to a high end-diastolic pressure and can therefore lead to pulmonary oedema.

It is highly unlikely that you will be presented with a patient who has HOCM to diagnose as a short case in finals, but you may be presented with such a patient as a long case. The signs (Fig. 20.2) to watch for are:

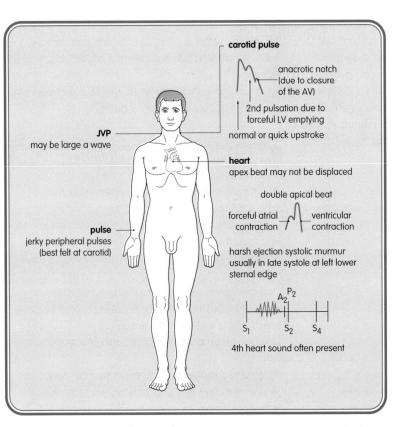

Fig. 20.2 Important clinical signs in hypertrophic obstructive cardiomyopathy. (AV, aortic valve; JVP, jugular venous pressure; LV, left ventricle.)

- Jerky peripheral pulse—the second rise palpable in the pulse is due to the rise in left ventricular pressure as the left ventricle attempts to overcome the outflow tract obstruction.
- Double apical beat—the stiff left ventricle causes raised left ventricular end-diastolic pressure. The atrial contraction is therefore very forceful to fill the left ventricle. It is this atrial impulse that can be felt in addition to the left ventricular contraction that gives this classical sign.
- Systolic thrill—felt at the left lower sternal edge.
- Systolic murmur—crescendo and decrescendo in nature, and best heard between the apex and the left lower sternal edge.

It may be difficult to differentiate between HOCM and aortic stenosis on examination. Use the following features to help:

- Pulse—slow rising in aortic stenosis, jerky or with a normal upstroke in HOCM.
- Thrill and murmur—both found in the second right intercostal space in aortic stenosis and at the left lower sternal edge in HOCM.

- Variation of the murmur with Valsalva manoeuvre—this does not occur in aortic stenosis, but the murmur of HOCM is increased because the volume of the left ventricle is reduced by the manoeuvre and therefore the outflow obstruction worsens.

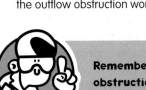

Remember that the outflow obstruction of aortic stenosis is fixed and is present throughout systole whereas the obstruction of HOCM is often absent at the start of systole and worsens as the ventricle empties.

Diagnosis and investigations
Electrocardiography
This is usually abnormal in HOCM. The most common abnormalities are T wave and ST segment abnormalities, the signs of left ventricular hypertrophy may also be present.

Continuous ambulatory electrocardiography

The presence of ventricular arrhythmias is common in patients who have HOCM and is a cause of sudden death. It is thought that the presence of ventricular arrhythmias on an ambulatory ECG monitor is a risk factor for sudden death and that an antiarrhythmic agent should be commenced. These tests are usually performed as part of a yearly screening programme for these patients.

Echocardiography

This is the most useful investigation because it confirms the diagnosis and can be used to assess the degree of outflow tract obstruction.

Characteristic echocardiography findings include:
- Asymmetric hypertrophy of the septum.
- Abnormal systolic anterior motion of the anterior leaflet of the mitral valve.
- Left ventricular outflow tract obstruction.

Prognosis

Children who are diagnosed when they are under 14 years of age have a poor prognosis and a high incidence of sudden death. Adults have a better prognosis, but they also have a higher mortality rate than the general population. Another outcome is progressive cardiac failure with cardiac dilatation.

Management

Drug management

As with aortic stenosis, vasodilators should be avoided because they worsen the gradient across the obstruction. Therefore patients who have HOCM should not receive nitrates.

β-Blockers (β-adrenoceptor antagonists) are used because their negative inotropic effect acts to decrease the contractility of the hypertrophied septum and reduce the outflow tract obstruction.

Antiarrhythmic agents are important in patients who have ventricular and atrial arrhythmias. Patients who have atrial fibrillation should be cardioverted as soon as possible (patients who have a high left ventricular end-diastolic pressure rely on the atrial impulse to fill the left ventricle effectively).

Dual chamber pacing

This reduces the outflow tract gradient by pacing the heart from the right ventricular apex and therefore altering the pattern of septal motion.

Surgery

Surgery is used only when all other treatments have failed. A myomectomy is performed on the abnormal septum.

There is a new catheter technique to infarct the septum by occluding the septal artery.

RESTRICTIVE CARDIOMYOPATHY

This is the least common of the cardiomyopathies in developed countries.

The ventricular walls are excessively stiff and impede ventricular filling; therefore end-diastolic pressure is increased. The systolic function of the ventricle is often normal.

Presentation is identical to that of constrictive pericarditis, but the two must be differentiated because pericarditis is treatable with surgery.

Possible causes of restrictive cardiomyopathy include:
- Storage diseases (e.g. glycogen storage diseases).
- Infiltrative diseases (e.g. amyloidosis, sarcoidosis).
- Scleroderma.
- Endomyocardial diseases (e.g. endomyocardial fibrosis, hypereosinophilic syndrome, carcinoid).

Note that if amyloid is found on endomyocardial biopsy or if the patient has been clearly diagnosed with haemachromatosis or scleroderma then the disorder cannot technically be called a cardiomyopathy because the cause is known.

Clinical features

The main features are:
- Dyspnoea and fatigue due to poor cardiac output.
- Peripheral oedema and ascites.
- Elevated jugular venous pressure with a positive Kussmaul's sign (increase in jugular venous pressure during inspiration).

Management

There is no specific treatment and the condition usually progresses towards death relatively quickly; most patients do not survive 10 years after diagnosis.

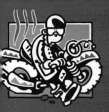

21. Pericarditis and Pericardial Effusion

The pericardium forms a strong protective sac around the heart. It is composed of an outer fibrous and an inner serosal layer with approximately 50 ml of pericardial fluid between these in the healthy state.

ACUTE PERICARDITIS

Acute pericarditis is caused by inflammation of the pericardium (Fig. 21.1).

Clinical features
History
The chest pain of acute pericarditis is usually central or left-sided pain that is sharp in nature and relieved by sitting forwards. Aggravating factors include lying supine and coughing.

Dyspnoea may be caused by the pain of deep inspiration or the haemodynamic effects of an associated pericardial effusion.

On examination
The patient may have a fever and tachycardia.

A pericardial friction rub may be heard on auscultation of the heart. This is a high-pitched scratching sound (therefore heard best with the diaphragm). It characteristically varies with time and may appear and disappear from one examination to the next. It sounds closer to the ears than a murmur.

Investigation
Blood tests
These will provide evidence of active inflammation—raised white cell count, erythrocyte sedimentation rate (ESR), and C-reactive protein (CRP), and also clues about the underlying cause.

The following blood tests are appropriate:
- Full blood count.
- ESR and CRP.
- Urea, creatinine, and electrolytes.
- Viral titres in the acute and convalescent phase (3 weeks later); also urine and faecal samples for viral studies and a Paul–Bunnell test.
- Blood cultures (at least three).
- Autoantibody titres (e.g. antinuclear antibodies, rheumatoid factor).
- Cardiac enzymes.

Fig. 21.1 Causes of acute pericarditis. (HIV, human immunodeficiency virus; MI, myocardial infarction; SLE, systemic lupus erythematosus.)

Causes of acute pericarditis	
Cause	Examples/comment
viral infection	coxsackievirus A and B, echovirus, Epstein–Barr virus, HIV
bacterial infection	pneumococci, staphylococci, Gram-negative organisms, *Neisseria meningitidis, N. gonorrhoeae*
fungal infection	histoplasmosis, candidal infection
other infections	tuberculosis
acute MI	occurs in up to 25% of patients 12 hours–6 days after infarction
uraemia	usually a haemorrhagic pericarditis and may rapidly lead to cardiac tamponade; uraemic pericarditis is an indication for haemodialysis
autoimmune disease	acute rheumatic fever, SLE, rheumatoid arthritis, scleroderma
other causes	neoplastic disease, other inflammatory diseases (e.g. sarcoidosis, Whipple's disease, Behçet's syndrome, Dressler's syndrome (i.e. post-cardiotomy syndrome)

Electrocardiography

Superficial myocardial injury caused by pericarditis results in characteristic ECG changes (Fig. 21.2).

- Concave ST segment elevation is usually present in all leads except AVR and V1.
- Subsequently a few days later the ST segments return to normal and T wave flattening occurs and may even become inverted.
- Finally all of the changes resolve and the ECG trace returns to normal (this may take several weeks or if the inflammation persists may remain for many months).

A dissecting thoracic aortic aneurysm may occasionally present as acute pericarditis or a pericardial effusion. Therefore be careful to look for a widened mediastinum of the chest radiograph and if this is suspicious a computed tomography scan of the chest should be performed to avoid missing this diagnosis.

Chest radiography

This is normal in most cases of uncomplicated acute pericarditis; however, a number of changes are possible:

- A pericardial effusion may develop and if large will result in enlargement of the cardiac shadow, which assumes a globular shape.
- Pleural effusions may also be seen.

Echocardiography

This is the best investigation for confirming the presence of a pericardial effusion. In uncomplicated acute pericarditis, however, echocardiography may be normal.

Management

Any treatable underlying cause should of course be sought and treated appropriately. Most cases of pericarditis are viral or idiopathic. The main aims of management are therefore analgesia and bed rest. Non-steroidal anti-inflammatory agents are the most effective for this condition. Occasionally a short course of oral corticosteroids is required.

A pericardial effusion may be present. If large or causing tamponade this can be drained. Analysis of the effusion may provide clues about the underlying cause of the pericarditis.

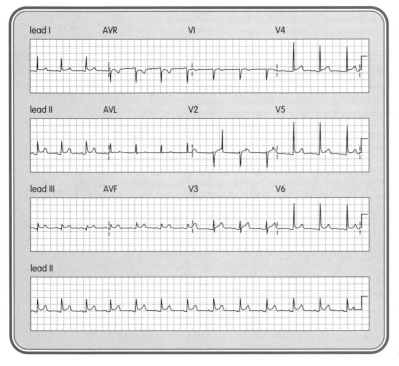

Fig. 21.2 ECG changes of pericarditis. Note the concave or saddle-shaped ST elevation seen in all leads except AVR.

DRESSLER'S SYNDROME

Dressler's syndrome is a syndrome of fever, pericarditis, and pleurisy occurring more than 1 week after a cardiac operation or myocardial infarction. It can only occur if the pericardium has been exposed to the blood. Antibodies form against the pericardial antigens and then attack the pericardium in a type III autoimmune reaction.

Patients present with fever, malaise, and chest pain. They exhibit the classic signs of acute pericarditis. They may also have arthritis. Cardiac tamponade is not uncommon.

Chest radiography shows pleural effusions. Echocardiography may reveal a pericardial effusion.

Management consists of non-steroidal anti-inflammatory agents and aspirin initially. Corticosteroids may be added if symptoms persist.

CHRONIC CONSTRICTIVE PERICARDITIS

Chronic constrictive pericarditis occurs when the pericardium becomes fibrosed and thickened and eventually restricts the filling of the heart during diastole. Causes are listed in Fig. 21.3.

Clinical features

The restricted filling of all four chambers of the heart results in low-output failure.

Initially the right-sided component is more marked resulting in a high venous pressure and hepatic congestion.

Later left ventricular failure becomes apparent with dyspnoea and orthopnoea.

Causes of chronic restrictive pericarditis

viral infection
tuberculosis
mediastinal radiotherapy
mediastinal malignancy
autoimmune disease

Fig. 21.3 Causes of chronic restrictive pericarditis. Note that any cause of acute pericarditis can persist and lead to chronic constrictive pericarditis. The diseases listed here, however, seem to be the most common causes.

On examination

On examination the signs of right and left ventricular failure are evident, but these ventricles are not enlarged.

The single most important feature in the examination of such a patient is the jugular venous pressure (JVP), which is elevated as expected. Kussmaul's sign—an increase in the JVP during inspiration—may be evident.

Another important feature of the JVP is a rapid x and y descent. This is an important differential diagnostic point when trying to exclude tamponade. There is no such feature in tamponade.

The heart sounds are often soft. Atrial fibrillation is common.

Investigation

Blood tests are carried out to exclude a possible underlying cause (e.g. leucocytosis in infection, viral titres).

On chest radiography the heart size is normal. There may be signs of a neoplasm or tuberculosis. Pleural effusions are not uncommon. Tuberculous pericarditis may be associated with radiographically visible calcification.

Echocardiography shows good left ventricular function.

Cardiac catheterization is diagnostic because it shows the classical pattern of raised left and right end-diastolic pressures with normal left ventricular function on the ventriculogram.

Management

The only definitive treatment is pericardectomy.

Antituberculous therapy may be required if the underlying cause is tuberculosis and should be continued for 1 year.

PERICARDIAL EFFUSION

A pericardial effusion is an accumulation of fluid in the pericardial space.

Cardiac tamponade describes the condition where a pericardial effusion increases the intrapericardial pressure.

Causes

Causes of pericardial effusion (Fig. 21.4) include:
- Acute pericarditis (see Fig. 21.1).
- Myocardial infarction with ventricular wall rupture.
- Chest trauma.

Causes of a pericardial effusion	
Type of effusion	**Examples**
transudate (<30 g/L protein)	congestive cardiac failure, hypoalbuminaemia
exudate (>30 g/L protein)	infection (viral, bacterial or fungal), post-myocardial infarction, malignancy (e.g. local invasion of lung tumour, systemic lupus erythematosus, Dressler's syndrome)
haemorrhagic	uraemia, aortic dissection, trauma

Fig. 21.4 Causes of a pericardial effusion.

- Cardiac surgery.
- Aortic dissection.
- Anticoagulation.

Clinical features

A pericardial effusion may remain asymptomatic even if very large if it accumulates gradually. As much as 2 L of fluid can be accommodated without an increase in intrapericardial pressure if it accumulates slowly, but as little as 100 mL can cause tamponade if it appears suddenly.

History

The only symptoms produced by a large chronic effusion may be a dull ache in the chest or dysphagia from compression of the oesophagus.

If cardiac tamponade is present, however, the patient may complain of dyspnoea, abdominal swelling (due to ascites), and peripheral oedema.

Examination

The important examination findings in a patient who has tamponade are:
- Low blood pressure.
- Pulse—low volume, and may be pulsus paradoxus

(where there is an exaggerated reduction of the pulse >10 mmHg during inspiration).
- Soft heart sounds and rarely a pericardial rub.

Possible mechanisms for pulsus paradoxus
These are:
- Increased venous return during inspiration filling the right heart and restricting left ventricular filling because the pericardium forms a rigid sac with only limited space within it.
- Downward movement of the diaphragm causing traction on the pericardium and tightening it further (this theory is not widely supported).

Investigation
Electrocardiography
A pericardial effusion results in the production of small voltage complexes with variable axis (electrical alternans is caused by the movement of the heart within the fluid).

On chest radiography the heart may appear large and globular.

Echocardiography reveals the pericardial effusion. Right ventricular diastolic collapse is a classical echocardiographic sign of tamponade.

Management
The pericardial effusion should be drained.

If the patient is in cardiogenic shock due to tamponade an emergency pericardial needle aspiration may be performed followed by formal drainage once the patient has been resuscitated.

Either technique involves insertion of the drain or needle just below the xiphisternum and advancing it at 45 degrees to the skin in the direction of the patient's left shoulder.

The fluid should be sent for cytology, microscopy, culture and biochemical analysis of protein content.

Long-term treatment depends upon the underlying cause.

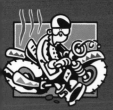

22. Valvular Heart Disease

This topic has been touched upon in Chapters 6 and 10, but it is covered here in more detail.

Valve lesions are a common short case question both in finals and in the membership examination. One way to learn valve disease in to learn it parrot fashion; once you know it you will not forget it again so it will be time well spent (Fig. 22.1). Alternatively, familiarity with the physiology (see *Crash Course: Cardiovascular System* by R. Sunthareswaran) will enable you to understand the features of valve disease from first principles.

RHEUMATIC FEVER

As mentioned in Chapter 23, rheumatic fever is much less common in the developed world than in developing countries due to better social conditions and antibiotic therapy, and also because of a reduction in the virulence of β-haemolytic streptococcus. It is still a major problem in the developing world where it is responsible for more heart disease than any other single disease.

Causes

Rheumatic fever is caused by a group A streptococcal pharyngeal infection. It occurs 2–3 weeks later in a small percentage of children aged 5–15 years. It is an antibody-mediated autoimmune response and occurs where antibodies directed against bacterial cell membrane antigens cross-react and cause multiorgan disease.

Clinical features

Diagnosis is entirely clinical. Diagnosis based on the Duckett–Jones criteria requires evidence of preceding β-haemolytic streptococcal infection (e.g. increased antistreptolysin O titres) plus one major criterion or two minor criteria. Major criteria are:

- Carditis—involves all layers (pancarditis) and is usually asymptomatic.
- Arthritis—a migrating polyarthritis affecting the larger joints.
- Sydenham's chorea—usually occurs months after the initial disease and characterized by involuntary movements of the face and mouth due to inflammation of the caudate nucleus.
- Erythema marginatum—seen mainly on the trunk; the rash has raised red edges and a clear centre and the shape of the lesions changes with time.
- Nodules—pea sized subcutaneous nodules on the extensor surfaces (painless).

Minor criteria are:

- Fever.
- Previous rheumatic fever.
- Raised erythrocyte sedimentation rate (ESR) or C-reactive protein (CRP).
- Long PR interval.
- Arthralgia.

Investigations

Blood tests reveal raised inflammatory markers (ESR and CRP) and rising antistreptolysin O (ASO) titres when taken 2 weeks apart. The throat swab may be positive.

Management

Treatment with high-dose benzylpenicillin is started immediately to eradicate the causative organism. Anti-inflammatory agents are given to suppress the autoimmune response. Salicylates are effective. Corticosteroids are used if there is any carditis.

Valve lesions and their abbreviations	
Valve involved	**Lesion**
mitral valve	mitral stenosis (MS) mitral regurgitation (MR) floppy (prolapsing) mitral valve (MVP)
aortic valve	aortic stenosis (AS) aortic regurgitation (AR)
tricuspid valve	tricuspid regurgitation (TR) tricuspid stenosis (TS)
pulmonary valve	pulmonary stenosis (PS) pulmonary regurgitation (PR)

Fig. 22.1 Valve lesions and their abbreviations.

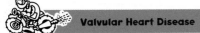

Long-term follow-up is required and any patients who have resulting valve damage need prophylactic antibiotics to prevent infective endocarditis.

Acute rheumatic fever is extremely uncommon in the developed world, but it is a good idea to have an idea of this disease because there are still many elderly people who have the after-effects of the disease. It is also important to recognize and treat acute rheumatic fever promptly.

MITRAL STENOSIS

Causes

The most common cause of mitral stenosis (MS) is rheumatic fever (Fig. 22.2). Other causes are:
- Congenital (Lutembacher's syndrome—MS associated with an atrial septal defect).

- Malignant—carcinoid (rare).
- Systemic lupus erythematosus.
- Left atrial myxoma.

Rheumatic fever causes fusion of the cusps and commissures and thickening of the cusps, which then become immobile and stenosed in a fish-mouth configuration[2]. An immobile valve often cannot close properly and is therefore often regurgitant as well.

Clinical features

The main presenting features of MS are:
- Dyspnoea—this may be due to pulmonary hypertension or pulmonary oedema. Patients who have MS have an increased incidence of chest infections, which may cause dyspnoea.
- Haemoptysis—there is an increased incidence of pulmonary vein and alveolar capillary rupture.
- Palpitations—atrial fibrillation is common in this condition and may cause palpitations, which are often accompanied by a sudden worsening in the dyspnoea because the loss of the atrial contraction (upon which the heart has become dependent) causes a considerable reduction in cardiac output.
- Systemic emboli—a recognized complication of atrial fibrillation.

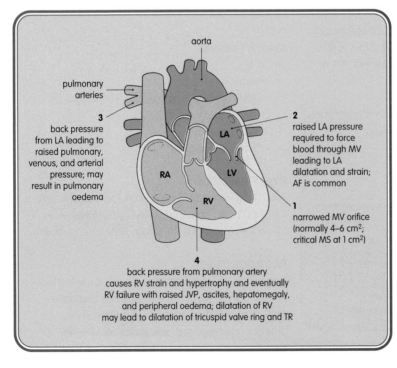

Fig. 22.2 Pathophysiology of mitral stenosis. (LA, left atrium; LV, left ventricle; JVP, jugular venous pressure; MV, mitral valve; RA, right atrium; RV, right ventricle; TR, tricuspid regurgitation.)

aorta

pulmonary arteries

3
back pressure from LA leading to raised pulmonary, venous, and arterial pressure; may result in pulmonary oedema

2
raised LA pressure required to force blood through MV leading to LA dilatation and strain; AF is common

LA

RA

LV

RV

1
narrowed MV orifice (normally 4–6 cm²; critical MS at 1 cm²)

4
back pressure from pulmonary artery causes RV strain and hypertrophy and eventually RV failure with raised JVP, ascites, hepatomegaly, and peripheral oedema; dilatation of RV may lead to dilatation of tricuspid valve ring and TR

Symptoms that are secondary to effects of left atrial enlargement include:

- Hoarseness due to stretching of the recurrent laryngeal nerve.
- Dysphagia due to oesophageal compression.
- Left lung collapse due to compression of the left main bronchus.

On examination

The principal clinical findings (Fig. 22.3) are:

- Loud first heart sound (S_1) due to the mitral valve slamming shut at the beginning of ventricular systole.
- A tapping apex beat that is not displaced.
- An opening snap after the second heart sound (S_2) followed by a low rumbling mid-diastolic murmur heard best at the apex with the patient on his or her left side and in expiration. If you have not listened in exactly this way you cannot exclude MS.
- If the patient is in sinus rhythm, the mid-diastolic murmur has a pre-systolic accentuation; this is absent if the patient has atrial fibrillation. Severity is related to the duration, not the intensity of the mid-diastolic murmur.
- If pulmonary hypertension has developed then the pulmonary component of the second heart sound (P_2) is loud and palpable and there may

be a right ventricular heave. Tricuspid regurgitation may be present.

Mitral stenosis is a difficult murmur to hear. It is therefore vital to listen for the murmur correctly (i.e. with the patient on his or her left side in full expiration). Unless you do this you cannot say you've excluded a diagnosis of mitral stenosis.

Investigations

Investigations that may aid diagnosis include the following.

Electrocardiography

Atrial fibrillation may be seen. P mitrale is another feature and is only seen in sinus rhythm. The p wave in lead II is abnormally long (>0.12 s) and may have an 'M' shape.

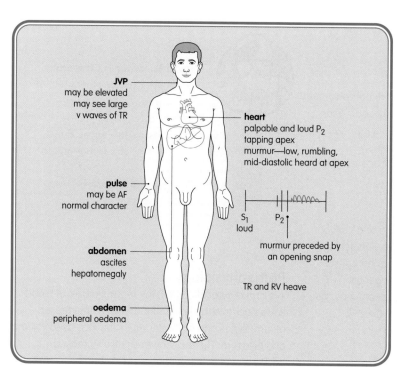

Fig. 22.3 Clinical findings in patients who have mitral stenosis. (AF, atrial fibrillation; S_1, first heart sound; P_2, pulmonary component of second heart sound.)

JVP
may be elevated
may see large
v waves of TR

heart
palpable and loud P_2
tapping apex
murmur—low, rumbling,
mid-diastolic heard at apex

pulse
may be AF
normal character

S_1
loud

P_2

murmur preceded by
an opening snap

abdomen
ascites
hepatomegaly

TR and RV heave

oedema
peripheral oedema

Chest radiography

This shows the enlarged left atrium. The carina may be widely split. The mitral valve itself may be calcified and therefore visible. There may be prominent pulmonary vessels.

Echocardiography

The mitral valve can be visualized and the cross-sectional area measured. Pulmonary hypertension can also be measured.

Cardiac catheterization

This is performed on most patients before valve replacement to exclude any coexistent coronary artery disease and evaluate any mitral regurgitation that may be present.

Management
Medical management

Medical treatment of MS may consist of:

- Digoxin or a small dose of a β-blocker (β-adrenoceptor antagonist)—may be used to treat atrial fibrillation. Direct current (DC) cardioversion may be successful in patients who have atrial fibrillation of recent onset, but only if they have been fully anticoagulated for at least 4 weeks.
- Anticoagulation with warfarin is recommended in all patients who have MS and atrial fibrillation.
- Diuretics are used to treat the pulmonary and peripheral oedema.

Surgical management

This is indicated in patients who have a mitral valve area of 1 cm^2 or less. Note that restenosis may occur after any valvuloplasty or valvotomy. In carefully selected patients this does not occur for many years, early restenosis within 5 years may occur in those who have thickened or rigid valves

Mitral valvuloplasty

Mitral valvuloplasty involves the passage of a balloon across the mitral valve and its inflation, so stretching the stenosed valve. This procedure is carried out via a percutaneous route and only requires a local anaesthetic and light sedation. The following features make a patient unsuitable for this procedure:

- Marked mitral regurgitation.
- A history of systemic emboli.
- Calcified or thickened rigid mitral valve leaflets.

Open mitral valvotomy

Open mitral valvotomy is performed under general anaesthetic using a median sternotomy incision and requires cardiopulmonary bypass. It is used in patients who have already had a mitral valvuloplasty or who have mild mitral regurgitation.

Closed mitral valvotomy

This has now been superceded by mitral valvuloplasty. It does not require cardiopulmonary bypass. A curved incision is made under the left breast. It is worth knowing this because patients in finals examinations may have this scar.

Mitral valve replacement

This is used for calcified or very rigid valves unsuitable for valvuloplasty or valvotomy.

MITRAL REGURGITATION

The mitral valve may become incompetent for four reasons (Fig. 22.4):

- Abnormal mitral valve annulus.
- Abnormal mitral valve leaflets.
- Abnormal chordae tendinae.
- Abnormal papillary muscle function.

When considering the causes of regurgitation of any valve it is useful to divide the causes into:

- Abnormalities of the valve ring.
- Abnormalities of the valve cusps and leaflets.
- Abnormalities of the supporting structures.

Pathophysiology

In mitral regurgitation (MR) the regurgitant jet of blood flows back into the left atrium and with time the left atrium dilates and accommodates the increased volume and pressure. There is, however, also increased backpressure in the pulmonary veins and as the MR

Causes of MR	
Site of pathology	Pathology
mitral annulus	senile calcification left ventricular dilatation and enlargement of the annulus abscess formation during infective endocarditis
mitral valve leaflets	infective endocarditis rheumatic fever prolapsing (floppy) mitral valve congenital malformation connective tissue disorders—Marfan syndrome, Ehlers–Danlos syndrome, ostoegenesis inperfecta, pseudoxanthoma elasticum
chordae tendinae	idiopathic rupture myxomatous degeneration infective endocarditis connective tissue disorders
papillary muscle	myocardial infarction infiltration—sarcoid, amyloid myocarditis

Fig. 22.4 Causes of mitral regurgitation.

worsens pulmonary hypertension develops, which may eventually cause right ventricular hypertrophy and failure.

The left ventricle is dilated, because the blood entering from the left atrium with each beat is increased; this results in left ventricular hypertrophy and may, if severe, cause left ventricular dilatation and failure. Severe, chronic MR will, if not treated, result in biventricular failure. (Mitral stenosis differs because it does not cause left ventricular failure.)

Clinical features

These vary depending upon whether the MR is chronic or acute:

- Chronic mitral regurgitation develops slowly so allowing the heart to compensate and usually presents with a history of fatigue and dyspnoea.
- Acute MR presents with severe dyspnoea due to pulmonary oedema. The left atrium has not had time to dilate to accommodate the increased volume due to regurgitation of blood back through the mitral valve. The pressure increase is therefore transmitted directly to the pulmonary veins, resulting in pulmonary oedema.

Acute MR can be rapidly fatal and needs to be looked for in patients following myocardial infarction (papillary muscle rupture occurs at days 4–7 after myocardial infarction) and in patients who have infective endocarditis.

On examination

Features that may be seen are illustrated in Fig. 22.5 and include the following:

- Atrial fibrillation—an irregularly irregular pulse is common, especially in patients who have chronic MR and a dilated left atrium.
- Jugular venous pressure may be elevated—if the patient has developed pulmonary hypertension and right heart failure, or fluid retention.
- The apex is displaced downward and laterally as the left ventricle dilates—eventually left ventricular failure may result. (Note that in MS the apex is not displaced because the left ventricle is protected by the stenosed mitral valve.)
- The murmur of MR is pansystolic and best heard at the apex. The murmur radiates to the axilla. Note that the loudness of the murmur is not an indicator of the severity of the MR.
- Signs of congestive cardiac failure (i.e. third heart sound, bilateral basal inspiratory crepitations, ascites, peripheral oedema).
- P_2 may be loud and there may be a right ventricular heave—if pulmonary hypertension has developed.

Floppy mitral valve

This is also known as the prolapsing mitral valve. Factors to consider are:

- This is a common disorder affecting approximately 4% of the population and more females than males.

169

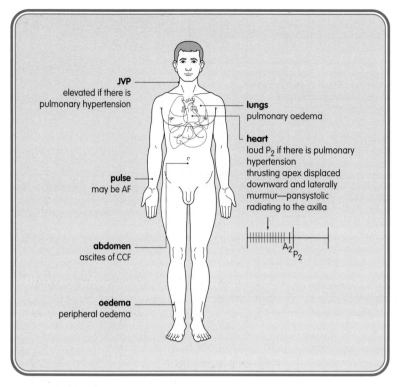

Fig. 22.5 Clinical findings in patients who have mitral regurgitation. (A₂, aortic component of second heart sound; AF, atrial fibrillation; CCF, congestive cardiac failure; P₂, pulmonary component of second heart sound.)

In the figure:

JVP elevated if there is pulmonary hypertension

lungs pulmonary oedema

heart loud P_2 if there is pulmonary hypertension thrusting apex displaced downward and laterally murmur—pansystolic radiating to the axilla

pulse may be AF

abdomen ascites of CCF

oedema peripheral oedema

- The mitral valve may merely prolapse minimally into the left atrium or cause varying degrees of MR.
- Most cases are idiopathic, but floppy mitral valve is seen with greater frequency in certain conditions (e.g. Marfan syndrome and other connective tissue disorders).
- Most patients are asymptomatic, the disorder being diagnosed at routine medical examination. Some patients present with fatigue, atypical chest pain, and palpitations.
- Examination reveals a mid-systolic click at the apex. This may or may not be followed by a systolic murmur of mitral regurgitation,
- Prophylaxis against infective endocarditis is only indicated in those patients who have MR.
- Most patients require no further treatment other than reassurance.

Investigations

The following investigations may aid diagnosis:

Electrocardiography

There may be atrial fibrillation and left ventricular hypertrophy.

Chest radiography

An enlarged left ventricle may be seen as an increase in the cardiothoracic ratio The mitral valve may be calcified and therefore visible

Echocardiography

The mitral valve can be clearly seen and the regurgitant jet visualized. The left atrium and ventricular sizes can be assessed.

Cardiac catheterization

Most patients have minimal MR on echocardiography and do not require catheterization. This is performed to assess the severity of the MR and to exclude other valve lesions and coronary artery disease.

Management

Medical management

This may consist of:

- Digoxin and anticoagulation and possibly triggered DC conversion for atrial fibrillation.
- Diuretics and angiotensin-converting enzyme inhibitors to treat the congestive cardiac failure.

Causes of AS	
Type of AS	**Cause**
valvular AS	congenital most common, males > females (deformed valve may be uni-, bi-, or tricuspid) senile calcification rheumatic fever severe atherosclerosis
subvalvular AS	fibromuscular ring HOCM
supravalvular AS	associated with hypercalcaemia in Williams syndrome, a syndrome associated with elfin facies, mental retardation, strabismus, hypervitaminosis D, and hypercalcaemia; the inheritance is autosomal dominant

Fig. 22.6 Causes of aortic stenosis. (HOCM, hypertrophic obstructive cardiomyopathy.)

Surgical management

Patients are considered for surgery if the MR is severe at echocardiography and cardiac catheterization. It is important to act before irreversible left ventricular damage has occurred.

Mitral valve repair
This may take the form of mitral annuloplasty, repair of a ruptured chordae, or repair of a mitral valve leaflet. These procedures are performed on patients who have mobile non-calcified and non-thickened valves.

Mitral valve replacement
This is performed if mitral valve repair is not possible. Both repair and replacement of the mitral valve require a median sternotomy incision and cardiopulmonary bypass.

myocardial blood supply from the coronary arteries is reduced (coronary artery flow occurs during diastole—see *Crash Course: Cardiovascular System* by R. Sunthareswaran).

Clinical features
Patients are often asymptomatic; however, a number of symptoms are characteristic of AS, including:
- Dyspnoea—may lead to orthopnoea and paroxysmal nocturnal dyspnoea as the left ventricle fails
- Angina—due to the increased myocardial work and reduced blood supply (the coronary arteries may be normal).
- Dizziness and syncope—especially on exertion.
- Sudden death.
- Systemic emboli.

AORTIC STENOSIS

The commonest form of aortic stenosis (AS) is valvular AS; however, aortic stenosis may also occur at the sub- or supravalvular level (Fig. 22.6).

Pathophysiology
The left ventricular outflow obstruction results in an increased left ventricular pressure. The left ventricle undergoes hypertrophy and more vigorous and prolonged contraction to overcome the obstruction and maintain an adequate cardiac output. Myocardial oxygen demand is increased, and because systole is prolonged diastole is shortened and therefore

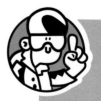

Patients who have aortic stenosis may present with angina, but an exercise test is absolutely contraindicated in patients who have severe aortic stenosis because even the mildest exertion can cause syncope or sudden death. Therefore it is crucial to examine every patient carefully before recommending an exercise ECG.

On examination

The following findings are common in valvular AS (Fig. 22.7):

- A slow rising, small volume pulse—best felt at the carotid pulse.
- A low blood pressure.
- Heaving apex beat—rarely displaced.
- Ejection systolic murmur at the aortic area radiating to the carotids accompanied by a palpable thrill.
- Signs of left ventricular or biventricular failure.

Investigations

Electrocardiography

This usually shows sinus rhythm and a picture of left ventricular hypertrophy with strain (tall R wave in lead V5 with deep S wave in lead V2 and T wave inversion in lateral leads).

Chest radiography

An enlarged cardiac shadow may occur due to left ventricular hypertrophy. The valve may be calcified and therefore visible. There may also be evidence of pulmonary oedema.

Echocardiography

This will show the valve in great detail including the number of cusps and their mobility and the presence of calcification. It will also show left ventricular hypertrophy or failure, and the aortic valve gradient can be measured using Doppler echocardiography.

Cardiac catheterization

This may provide information on the valve gradient and on left ventricular failure if not available from echocardiography. The coronary arteries are also assessed to rule out coronary artery disease that will require bypass grafting.

Management

Medical management

Apart from the use of diuretics to treat left ventricular failure, many antianginal drugs and angiotensin-converting enzyme inhibitors are avoided in AS because:

- They may have a negative inotropic effect and result in acute pulmonary oedema.
- They may vasodilate the patient, resulting in hypotension because the left ventricle is unable to compensate by increasing cardiac output.

Surgical management

This is considered in all symptomatic patients who have marked stenosis (aortic valve gradient >50 mmHg).

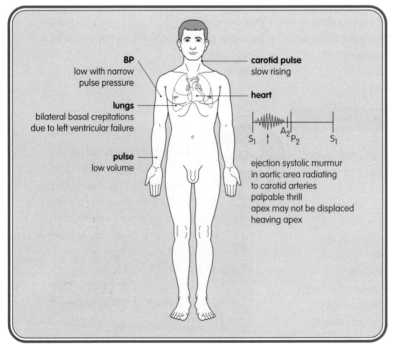

Fig. 22.7 Clinical findings in patients who have aortic stenosis.

Without operation the outcome for these patients is very poor.

Aortic valve replacement is usually performed using a median sternotomy incision and requires cardiopulmonary bypass

Aortic valvuloplasty is performed in children and rarely in the very elderly.

AORTIC REGURGITATION

Aortic regurgitation (AR) may be due to an abnormality of the valve cusps themselves or dilatation of the aortic root and therefore the valve ring (Fig. 22.8).

Pathophysiology
The regurgitation of blood back into the left ventricle after each systole results in an increased end-diastolic volume and an increased stroke volume. The left ventricle works harder and becomes hypertrophied. If the AR worsens the left ventricle may no longer be able to compensate and left ventricular failure will result. If the situation deteriorates further congestion results. The backpressure from the left ventricle may also cause pulmonary hypertension and right ventricular failure, but this is uncommon.

Clinical features
Moderate and mild AR are often asymptomatic. Dyspnoea is the main presenting feature (Fig. 22.9).

Causes of AR	
Type of disease	Cause
valve disease	congenital rheumatic fever infective endocarditis rheumatoid arthritis SLE connective tissue disease (e.g. Marfan syndrome, pseudoxanthoma elasticum)
aortic root disease	Marfan syndrome osteogenesis imperfecta type A aortic dissection ankylosing spondylitis Reiter's syndrome psoriatic arthritis

Fig. 22.8 Causes of aortic regurgitation. (SLE, systemic lupus erythematosus.)

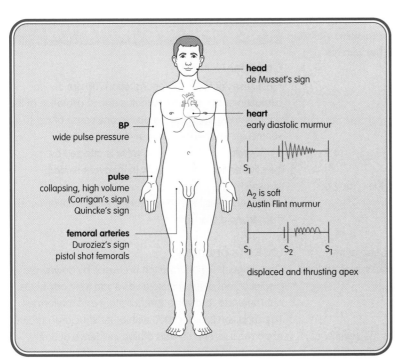

Fig. 22.9 Clinical findings in patients who have aortic regurgitation. (A_2, aortic component of second heart sound; S_1, first heart sound; S_2, second heart sound.)

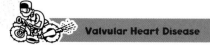

On examination

Characteristic findings in aortic regurgitation are:

- A collapsing high-volume pulse (waterhammer pulse)
  —due to the increased stroke volume and the rapid
  run-off of blood back into the left ventricle after
  systole. This is better felt at the carotid pulse, but
  can be felt at the radial pulse by lifting the arm and
  feeling the pulse with the fingers across it. The
  tapping quality is felt between the examiner's middle
  and distal interphalangeal joints.
- A wide pulse pressure on measuring blood pressure.
- Downward and laterally displaced apex, which has a
  thrusting nature.
- Murmur best heard at the left lower sternal edge with
  the patient sitting forward and in full expiration—it is
  a soft high-pitched early diastolic murmur, which is
  sometimes difficult to hear, so be sure to listen for it
  properly with a diaphragm.
- Increased flow across the aortic valve may produce
  an ejection systolic murmur.
- May be signs of left ventricular or biventricular
  failure.
- Other signs include De Musset's sign (head bobbing
  with each beat), Quincke's sign (visible capillary
  pulsation in the nailbed), pistol shot femoral pulses
  (an audible femoral sound) and Duroziez's sign
  (another audible murmur over the femoral arteries
  —a to and fro sound).
- The Austin Flint murmur heard when the regurgitant
  jet causes vibration of the anterior mitral valve leaflet.
  The murmur is similar to that of MS, but with no
  opening snap.

Investigations

Electrocardiography

This shows left ventricular hypertrophy.

Chest radiography

The left ventricle may be enlarged and there may be
pulmonary oedema

Echocardiography

The structure of the aortic valve and the size of the
regurgitant jet may be seen. Left ventricular function can
be assessed.

Cardiac catheterization

This is the most accurate way to assess the severity of
aortic regurgitation and also to assess the aortic root.

Left ventricular function can also be evaluated as can
the presence of coronary artery disease.

Management

Medical management

The use of diuretics and angiotensin-converting enzyme
inhibitors is valuable to treat cardiac failure in these
patients. It is, however, important to make the diagnosis
and surgically treat this condition before the left ventricle
dilates and fails.

Surgical management

This is considered if the patient is symptomatic or if
there are signs of progressive left ventricular dilatation.
The aortic root may also need to be replaced if it is
grossly dilated.

ASSESSING THE SEVERITY OF A VALVE LESION

Once a valve lesion has been diagnosed it is useful to
be able to comment on its severity. This is judged by
clinical, echocardiographic and angiographic means in
most cases (Fig. 22.10).

TRICUSPID REGURGITATION

Causes

Most cases of tricuspid regurgitation (TR) are due to
dilatation of the tricuspid annulus due to dilatation of the
right ventricle. This may be due to any cause of right
ventricular failure or pulmonary hypertension.

Occasionally the tricuspid valve is affected by
infective endocarditis (usually in intravenous drug
abusers).

Rarer causes include congenital malformations and
the carcinoid syndrome.

Ebstein's anomaly

This congenital malformation is caused by downward
displacement of the tricuspid valve into the body of the
right ventricle. The valve is regurgitant and malformed.
The condition is associated with other structural cardiac
abnormalities and there is a high incidence of both
supraventricular and ventricular tachyarrhythmias.

Features indicating severity of valve disease	
Valve disease	**Features**
MS	proximity of opening snap to second heart sound and duration of murmur valve area assessed on echocardiography evidence of pulmonary hypertension on echocardiography and cardiac catheterization
MR	symptoms and signs of pulmonary oedema size of regurgitant jet and poor left ventricular function on echocardiography evidence of pulmonary hypertension on echocardiography and cardiac catheterization
AS	presence of symptoms. low volume pulse and BP severity of aortic gradient and poor left ventricular function on echocardiography or cardiac catheterization
AR	signs of LVF left ventricular function and size of regurgitant jet at cardiac catheterization (echocardiography is useful but not as informative)

Fig. 22.10 Features indicating severity of valve disease. (AS, aortic stenosis; AR, aortic regurgitation; BP, blood pressure; LVF, left ventricular failure; MS, mitral stenosis; MR, mitral regurgitation.)

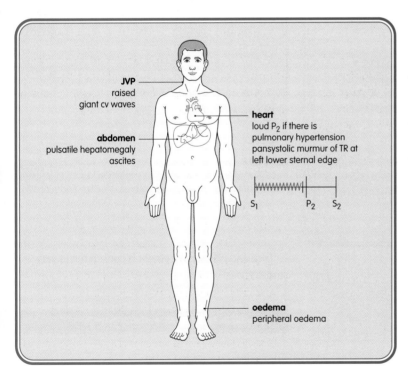

Fig. 22.11 Clinical findings in patients who have tricuspid regurgitation. Look out for signs of the underlying cause of right heart failure such as mitral valve disease or pulmonary disease. (JVP, jugular venous pressure; P_2, pulmonary component of second heart sound; S_1, first heart sound; S_2, second heart sound.)

Clinical features

The symptoms and signs are due to the backpressure effects of the regurgitant jet into the right atrium, which are transmitted to the venous system causing a prominent v wave in the jugular venous waveform (Fig. 22.11).

Fatigue and discomfort due to ascites or hepatic congestion are the commonest feature. Patients usually present with symptoms of the disease causing the underlying right ventricular failure; the TR is often an incidental finding.

175

Overview of other valve lesions			
Valve lesion	Cause	Clinical features	Management
tricuspid stenosis	rheumatic fever; rare	venous congestion—JVP raised, large a waves, ascites, hepatomegaly, peripheral oedema, soft diastolic murmur at left lower sternal edge	treat pulmonary hypertension, valve replacement
pulmonary stenosis	congenital malformation—Noonan's syndrome, maternal rubella syndrome, carcinoid syndrome	if mild asymptomatic, if severe—RVF and cyanosis, ejection systolic murmur in the pulmonary area (2nd left ICS), wide splitting of second heart sound	pulmonary valvuloplasty or pulmonary valve replacement
pulmonary regurgitation (PR)	dilatation of the valve ring secondary to pulmonary hypertension, infective endocarditis	RVF in severe cases, low pitched diastolic murmur in pulmonary area, Graham Steell murmur—in severe PR the murmur is high pitched due to the forceful jet and best heard at the left parasternal edge (i.e. similar to that in AR, but with signs of severe pulmonary hypertension and RVF)	treat underlying disease

Fig. 22.12 Overview of other valve lesions. (ICS, intercostal space; JVP, jugular venous pressure; RVF, right ventricular failure.)

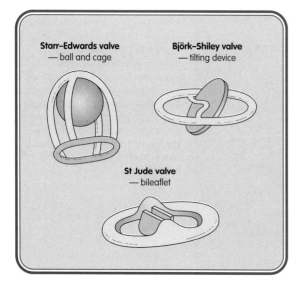

Fig. 22.13 Types of mechanical heart valve. Note that all patients must be anticoagulated for life and the international normalized ratio (INR) must be kept at approximately 3–4 —this lowers the risk of thromboembolism. They last for about 15 years. All patients who have prosthetic valves require antibiotic prophylaxis against infective endocarditis.

Types of biological heart valve	
Type of valve	Features
xenograft	manufactured from porcine valve or pericardium and mounted on a frame (on chest X-ray only the mounting ring can be seen) last for about 10 years
homograft	cadaveric valve graft more durable than a xenograft

Fig. 22.14 Types of biological heart valve. Anticoagulation is necessary only if the patient has atrial fibrillation. All patients require antibiotic prophylaxis against infective endocarditis.

Tricuspid valve replacement is considered in very severe cases.

OTHER VALVE LESIONS

These are summarized in Fig. 22.12.

PROSTHETIC HEART VALVES

Examples of mechanical and biological heart valves are shown in Figs 22.13 & 22.14.

Management
The mainstay of management is medical with diuretics and angiotensin-converting enzyme inhibitors to treat the right ventricular failure and fluid overload.

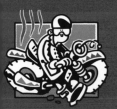

23. Infective Endocarditis

DEFINITION OF INFECTIVE ENDOCARDITIS

Infective endocarditis describes the condition where there is infection of the endothelial surface of the heart by a microorganism. Heart valves are most commonly affected, but any area causing a high-pressure jet through a narrow orifice may be involved (e.g. ventricular septal defect).

EPIDEMIOLOGY OF INFECTIVE ENDOCARDITIS

Infective endocarditis is an evolving disease. Traditionally the main predisposing condition was rheumatic fever; however, in developed countries rheumatic fever is much less common due to better social conditions and antibiotic therapy. Now in developed countries different groups of patients are presenting with infective endocarditis for the following reasons:

- Increased number of prosthetic valve insertions.
- Increased number of patients who have congenital heart disease surviving to adulthood.
- Increasing elderly population.
- Increasing intravenous drug abuse.
- Antibiotic resistance.

With this change in the population affected by infective endocarditis the organisms are also changing, for example coagulase-negative staphylococci, which were previously uncommon, are the most common organisms seen on prosthetic valves (Fig. 23.1).

Common causative organisms in infective endocarditis	
Organism	Comments
Streptococcus viridans group (i.e. S. milleri, S. mutans, S mitis)	still the most common causative organism; predominantly found on rheumatic heart valves or congenitally abnormal valves; can be found on prosthetic valves and in IVDAs
Staphylococcus aureus	most common cause in IVDAs; causes rapid destruction of the valve and there is a high mortality rate
coagulase-negative staphylococci (S. epidermidis)	most common cause in patients who have prosthetic heart valves within 2 months of operation (the high risk time for these patients); after 2 months the risk is much lower and other organisms may be involved
enterococci	can cause endocarditis in any situation and are probably the second most common causative organisms in developed countries
Gram-negative bacteria, diphtheroids	predominantly after valve surgery
fungi	IVDAs (Candida spp.) and after valve surgery
fastidious organisms (Gram-negative organisms requiring prolonged culture)	
Coxiella burnetii	

Fig. 23.1 Common causative organisms in infective endocarditis. Note that a significant number of cases are culture negative (i.e. grow no organism). (IVDAs, intravenous drug abusers.)

Conditions predisposing to infective endocarditis
rheumatic heart disease bicuspid aortic valve mitral valve prolapse with mitral regurgitation   (very rare in isolated mitral valve prolapse) ventricular septal defect patent ductus arteriosus prosthetic valves intravenous drug abuse (most commonly tricuspid valve) after myocardial infarct mural thrombus may become infected

Fig. 23.2 Conditions predisposing to infective endocarditis.

Conditions predisposing to transient bacteraemia

dental work—the most common cause; note that any type of
  dental work may give rise to it (even scaling)*
intravenous drug abuse
invasive procedures—intravenous cannulation, cystoscopy,*
  catheterization, surgery of any sort; any transrectal procedure*
bowel sepsis

Fig. 23.3 Conditions predisposing to transient bacteraemia. Note that upper gastrointestinal endoscopy is not thought to be a risk factor. *Procedures that are usually covered with prophylactic antibiotics.

People who have certain condions (Fig. 23.2) should be advised about the importance of antibiotic prophylaxis before certain procedures to prevent infective endocarditis. These procedures are as follows:

- Any dental work.
- Any operation.
- Any instrumentation of the urinary tract.
- Any transrectal procedure (e.g. prostatic biopsy, colonoscopy with biopsy).

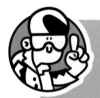

Oesophagogastro-duodenoscopy is not thought to require antibiotic prophylaxis. The antibiotics used for prophylaxis vary and advice should be sought from a microbiologist.

PATHOPHYSIOLOGY OF INFECTIVE ENDOCARDITIS

The development of endocarditis depends upon a number of factors:

- Presence of anatomical abnormalities in the heart surface.
- Haemodynamic abnormalities within the heart.
- Host immune response.
- Virulence of the organism.
- Presence of bacteraemia.

Transient bacteraemia is a common occurrence, but infective endocarditis is rare so a healthy individual

who has normal cardiac anatomy is well protected (Fig. 23.3).

Complications of infective endocarditis are potentially fatal and are as follows:

- Local destructive effects—valve incompetence, paravalvular abscesses, prosthetic valve dehiscence, and myocardial rupture. If they progress the local effects lead to congestive cardiac failure and cardiogenic shock; sometimes this is very rapid.
- Embolization of infected or non-infected fragments —these can result in stroke or cerebral abscess, ischaemic bowel, digital infarcts, renal and hepatic abscesses, renal infarcts (hepatic infarcts are rare because the liver is supplied by the hepatic artery and the hepatic portal system).
- Type III autoimmune reaction to the organism— resulting in the deposition of immune complexes (antibody plus antigen) and a subsequent inflammatory response. A diffuse or focal glomerulonephritis and arthritis may occur as a result.

If you remember these three classes of complications of infective endocarditis it is easy to fit actual symptoms and signs into each category. To classify signs according to the pathophysiology shows that you have a full understanding of the disease process and is bound to impress examiners.

CLINICAL FEATURES OF INFECTIVE ENDOCARDITIS

History

The duration of the symptoms is variable from a few days to several months. This tends to reflect the virulence of the organism—*Staphylococcus aureus* causes rapid valvular destruction and presents early whereas a *Staph. epidermidis* infection of a prosthetic valve may take a few months to present.

The following symptoms are common:

- Fever.
- Sweats.
- Anorexia and weight loss.
- General malaise.

Stroke is also seen as a presenting complaint, or myalgia and arthralgia. Important information to obtain from the patient for clues about the causative organism includes:

- A detailed history of any dental work, operations, or infections.
- Any history of rheumatic fever.
- Any history of intravenous drug abuse.

It is also important to find out about any drug allergies because long-term intravenous antibiotics may be needed.

On examination

A thorough examination is vital because it is sometimes possible to make the diagnosis on examination alone, which allows therapy to be started promptly. Failure to make the diagnosis early may have disastrous consequences because it is not uncommon to see this disease causing rapid valve destruction and cardiogenic shock.

A full examination is required because the signs occur in all systems (Fig. 23.4).

The following signs are characteristic of infective endocarditis:

- A murmur—the heart murmur is usually that of an incompetent valve because the infection often prevents the valve from closing either due to perforation of the valve leaflets or vegetations and adhesions impeding valve movement. It is important to perform daily cardiac auscultation because the murmur may change due to progressive valve

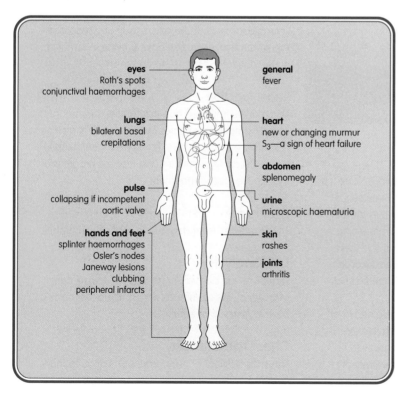

eyes
Roth's spots
conjunctival haemorrhages

general
fever

lungs
bilateral basal
crepitations

heart
new or changing murmur
S_3—a sign of heart failure

abdomen
splenomegaly

pulse
collapsing if incompetent
aortic valve

urine
microscopic haematuria

hands and feet
splinter haemorrhages
Osler's nodes
Janeway lesions
clubbing
peripheral infarcts

skin
rashes

joints
arthritis

Fig. 23.4 Important clinical findings in patients who have infective endocarditis.

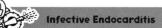

damage; this warns of imminent valve failure and an urgent echocardiogram is then necessary to evaluate the degree of valvular incompetence. The murmur of mitral regurgitation becomes louder as the regurgitation gets worse. The murmur of aortic regurgitation also gets louder and longer.

- Splenomegaly—a common finding especially if the history is long.
- Clubbing—develops after a few weeks of infective endocarditis. Other causes of clubbing include, cyanotic congenital heart disease, suppurative lung disease, squamous cell carcinoma of the lung, and inflammatory bowel disease.
- Splinter haemorrhages—more than four is pathological (remember that the most common cause of these is trauma).
- Osler's nodes and Janeway lesions—represent peripheral emboli (possibly septic).
- Roth's spots—retinal haemorrhages with a pale centre.
- Evidence of congestive cardiac failure.
- Microscopic haematuria on urine dipstick—always ask to dipstick the urine if you suspect infective endocarditis. This is a very sensitive test and easily carried out.
- Also peripheral emboli, features of a cerebrovascular event, inflamed joints.

When taking blood cultures it is important to maintain a good aseptic technique to minimize the risk of contaminating the samples. Clean the skin with iodine-containing skin wash (or the equivalent if the patient has iodine allergy). Take the blood and then inject it into the culture bottles, preferably using new needles.

INVESTIGATION OF A PATIENT WHO HAS INFECTIVE ENDOCARDITIS

Blood tests
Blood cultures

These are the most important investigations. Note the plural has been used because at least three sets of cultures must be performed. If possible they should be taken at least 1 hour apart before commencing antibiotic therapy. (If the patient is very ill and there is a high index of suspicion of infective endocarditis it is appropriate to start antibiotics after the first set has been obtained.)

Positive blood cultures are usually obtained in at least 95% cases of bacterial endocarditis if taken before antibiotic therapy. This allows therapy to be specifically directed according to the sensitivity of the organism.

Full blood count
Anaemia of chronic disease is common in patients who have less acute presentations. Other findings can include:

- Leucocytosis—may be seen as a sign of inflammation (usually a neutrophilia).
- Thrombocytopenia—may be an indication of disseminated intravascular coagulopathy.
- Thrombophilia—may be seen as part of the acute phase response.

Erythrocyte sedimentation rate and C-reactive protein
These are elevated as signs of inflammation. They are valuable markers of disease activity and repeated measurements every few days provide information on the patient's response to treatment.

Renal function
This may be impaired due to infarction or immune complex-mediated glomerulonephritis. This also needs repeating every few days during treatment as both aminoglycoside antibiotics and disease progression may cause renal impairment.

Liver function tests
These may be deranged due to septic microemboli.

Urinanalysis
As well as the bedside urine dipstick, formal urine microscopy should be performed to look for casts as seen in glomerulonephritis.

Chest radiography
This may be clear or may show signs of pulmonary oedema.

Echocardiography

Transthoracic echocardiography will reveal any valve incompetence and may also identify vegetations on the valve. This test is not very sensitive and cannot be used to exclude small vegetations.

Transoesophageal echocardiography is over 90% sensitive in diagnosing vegetations.

Remember that echocardiography is not a diagnostic test in infective endocarditis. It may help confirm the diagnosis and give information about the severity of the valve damage, but blood cultures are the only specific diagnostic test of infective endocarditis.

MANAGEMENT OF INFECTIVE ENDOCARDITIS

There are two main aims in the management of infective endocarditis:

- To effectively treat the infection with appropriate antibiotics with the minimum of drug-related complications.
- To diagnose and treat complications of the endocarditis (i.e. congestive cardiac failure, severe valve incompetence, peripheral abscesses, renal failure, etc.).

Antibiotic therapy

If infective endocarditis is suspected, antibiotic therapy is started as soon as the blood cultures have been taken (Fig. 23.5). The choice of agent can then be modified once the organism is known:

Intravenous therapy is used initially in all cases. This may be via the central or peripheral route. It is vital that the intravenous access sites are changed regularly to prevent infection (peripheral lines every 3 days, non-tunnelled central lines every 5–7 days). The sites should be inspected regularly and the line removed immediately if there is evidence of local infection.

Choice of antibiotic regimen

A microbiologist is the best person to decide what the antibiotic regimen should be and all cases of infective endocarditis should be reported to the microbiologist as soon as possible, even if blood cultures are negative.

Duration of antibiotic therapy

This depends upon the organism and the clinical response to treatment. Most bacterial infections require at least 6 weeks of intravenous therapy, although some centres change to oral therapy after 2 weeks if the response is good. The most important thing to remember is that the patient must be closely monitored after changing to oral therapy and after stopping therapy. If there is any evidence of recurrent disease activity intravenous therapy should be recommended.

Monitoring antibiotic therapy

Blood should be taken for:

- Antibiotic levels (gentamicin, vancomycin).
- To calculate the minimum inhibitory concentration (MIC)—the MIC gives an indication of the sensitivity of the organism to the antibiotics used. If it is not satisfactory another antimicrobial may be added.

Suggested antibiotic regimens		
Organism	Suggested agents	Adverse effects
Streptococcus viridans	benzylpenicillin 2.4 g IV 4-hourly (usually a 6-week course) and gentamicin	allergic reactions; penicillin—interstitial nephritis; gentamicin—8th cranial nerve and renal toxicity
Staphylococcus epidermidis	benzylpenicillin or flucloxacillin IV; fucidic acid may be added	fucidic acid—vomiting and hepatotoxicity
Staph. aureus	flucloxacillin and fucidic acid IV; gentamicin may also be useful initially	
Gram-negative organisms	ampicillin and gentamicin IV (dose according to levels)	
yeasts	flucytosine or amphotericin B	flucytosine—marrow depression and hepatic failure; amphotericin—renal failure

Fig. 23.5 Suggested antibiotic regimens. (IV, intravenously.)

181

In addition to antibiotic therapy the source of infection should be sought—the patient needs a thorough dental examination and any infected teeth removed because this is a common cause of recurrent bacteraemia. Similarly recurrent urinary tract infections should be prevented with prophylactic antibiotics.

COMPLICATIONS OF INFECTIVE ENDOCARDITIS

The following complications may occur:
- Congestive cardiac failure—the use of diuretics and angiotensin-converting enzyme inhibitors may be necessary. If cardiac failure remains severe due to profound valvular incompetence surgery to replace the valve is required.
- Thromboembolic complications—the use of anticoagulants is controversial; however, anticoagulation is used for patients who have thrombotic phenomena such as pulmonary embolus or deep venous thrombosis. Patients who have metal prosthetic valves should remain on their anticoagulation. Patients who have cerebral or peripheral arterial emboli are not anticoagulated because there is a risk of haemorrhage into the infarct.

MONITORING OF PATIENTS WHO HAVE INFECTIVE ENDOCARDITIS

This should include:
- Daily examination—this is the most important—look for worsening valvular incompetence, cardiac failure, new splinter hemorrhages, Roth's spots, Osler's nodes, etc., all suggestive of ongoing active disease.
- Temperature chart—an increase in temperature after the patient has been apyrexial for some time can represent reactivation of the infection and blood cultures should be sent immediately.
- Daily urine dipstick for microscopic haematuria—this is representative of disease activity.
- Twice weekly blood tests for full blood count, renal function, erythrocyte sedimentation rate, C-reactive protein, and liver function.

Indications for valve replacement in infective endocarditis
significant aortic or mitral regurgitation despite prolonged antibiotic therapy
persistent infection despite prolonged antibiotic therapy
large vegetations—these have a high incidence of embolization and can obstruct the valve orifice
aortic root abscess
unstable prosthetic valve (usually affects the sewing ring around prosthetic valves resulting in a perivalvular leak and occasionally dehiscence of the valve—this is an extremely dangerous condition and patients who have a significant perivalvular leak should be considered for valve replacement)

Fig. 23.6 Indications for valve replacement in infective endocarditis.

- Weekly ECG—look for lengthening of the PR interval. If an abscess develops around the aortic root or in the septum this affects the atrioventricular node and may lead to complete heart block.
- Weekly echocardiography—to assess vegetation size if they are visible, but more importantly to assess left ventricular function and the severity of the valve incompetence.

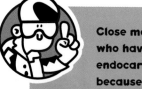

Close monitoring of patients who have infective endocarditis is crucial because any deterioration can lead to catastrophic valve incompetence if missed.

Operative intervention in active infective endocarditis carries a high mortality rate and marked morbidity. Indications for replacement of the infected valve are listed in Fig. 23.6. The patient should receive a full course of intravenous antibiotic treatment (at least 6 weeks) postoperatively.

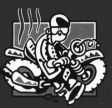

24. Hypertension

Hypertension is a major risk factor for cerebrovascular disease, myocardial infarction, cardiac failure, peripheral vascular disease and renal failure. To reduce the risk of these it is important to diagnose and adequately treat hypertensive patients.

DEFINITION OF HYPERTENSION

Normal blood pressure increases with age and varies throughout the day according to factors such as stress and exertion. There is also an underlying diurnal variation with the lowest blood pressure occurring at around 4 a.m.

The definition of hypertension therefore is that level of blood pressure associated with an increased risk of complications.

This equates to a level above 140/90 mmHg in adults.

CAUSES OF HYPERTENSION

Over 95% cases of hypertension are idiopathic and this is termed essential hypertension.

Secondary causes of hypertension, although rare are important to exclude because they may be curable (Fig. 24.1).

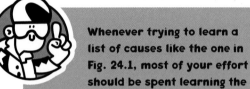

Whenever trying to learn a list of causes like the one in Fig. 24.1, most of your effort should be spent learning the main headings in the first column. Once you know these you will find your memory is triggered and you'll be able to recall at least two conditions for each category.

Causes of secondary hypertension	
Classification of cause	**Examples**
renal	renovascular disease, renal parenchymal diseases (e.g. polycystic kidney disease, glomerulonephritis, diabetic nephropathy—basically any significant renal disease), renin-producing tumours
endocrine	adrenal—Cushing's syndrome, congenital adrenal hyperplasia, Conn's syndrome, phaeochromocytoma acromegaly carcinoid hyper- or hypothyroidism oral contraceptive pill
vascular	coarctation of the aorta
drugs	oral contraceptive pill, corticosteroids, monoamine oxidase inhibitors
pregnancy	pregnancy-induced hypertension
neurological	increased intracranial pressure, sleep apnoea, acute porphyria, Guillain–Barré syndrome (may be associated with very large swings in blood pressure and heart rate)
alcohol	a common cause (alcohol intake is an important part of the history)

Fig 24.1 Causes of secondary hypertension. Whenever trying to learn a list of causes like this one most of your effort should be spent learning the main headings (i.e. classification)—you'll find that this will trigger your memory and you'll be able to recall at least two conditions for each category.

CLINICAL FEATURES OF HYPERTENSION

These are described in Chapter 7 and will not be repeated word for word here. The following is a summary of the clinical features of hypertension.

History

Most patients are entirely asymptomatic, but the presenting complaint may be headache, dizziness, or fainting.

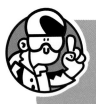

There is no correlation between symptoms and severity of hypertension in the vast majority of patients.

When checking the past medical history, ask about other risk factors for ischaemic heart disease such as:
- Smoking.
- Diabetes mellitus.
- Hypercholesterolaemia.
- Family history of heart disease.

Also be aware of the following:
- Evidence of cerebrovascular disease (cerebrovascular accident) or myocardial infarction in the past.
- If the patient is young think about possible secondary causes (e.g. recurrent urinary tract infections).

When checking the drug history, ask about all current medications including proprietary analgesics and the oral contraceptive pill.

With regards to the family history:
- Ask about family history of hypertension.
- If the patient is young think about possible secondary causes (e.g. family history of renal problems or cerebrovascular disease in polycystic kidney disease).

An assessment of social history should take into account:
- Smoking.
- Alcohol intake.
- Level of stress at work.
- Likelihood of non-compliance with medication.

On examination

Hypertension is diagnosed after three readings over 140/90 mmHg have been taken on separate occasions over a period of at least 3 months. Severe hypertension (e.g. >200/100 mmHg does not require three such readings for diagnosis).

Fig. 24.2 shows the important features to note on examination of a patient who has hypertension. Remember to look for signs of end-organ damage and signs of possible underlying causes of secondary hypertension.

The following are examples of end-organ damage secondary to hypertension:
- Ischaemic heart disease.
- Cardiac failure.
- Left ventricular hypertrophy.
- Cerebrovascular disease.
- Peripheral vascular disease.
- Renal impairment.
- Hypertensive retinopathy.

INVESTIGATION OF A PATIENT WHO HAS HYPERTENSION

Investigations, as listed in Fig. 24.3, should be performed at presentation and repeated on a yearly basis as a measure of how well the hypertension is responding to treatment. For example, left ventricular hypertrophy should gradually regress once hypertension has been successfully controlled.

These investigations are also directed towards looking for evidence of end-organ damage and possible causes of secondary hypertension.

If the patient is at high risk of having secondary hypertension then further investigations are indicated. The criteria for excluding secondary hypertension are as follows:
- Under 35 years of age.
- Symptoms and signs of malignant hypertension (i.e. blood pressure >180/100 mmHg, grade 3 or 4 hypertensive retinopathy, cardiac failure at a young age).
- Symptoms of an underlying cause (e.g. phaeochromocytoma—sweating, dizzy spells, tachycardia).
- Signs of an underlying cause (e.g. differential blood pressure in both arms, hyperkalaemia in the absence of diuretics, Cushingoid appearance).

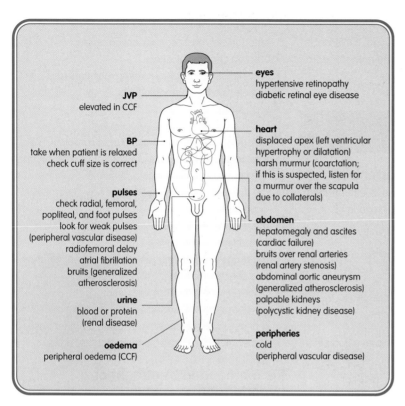

Fig. 24.2 Important clinical findings in hypertensive patients. Look for signs of end-organ damage and signs of the underlying cause of hypertension. It is essential to keep an open mind. This illustration is only a guide and there are many other possible findings (e.g. signs of thyroid disease or Cushing's syndrome). (CCF, congestive cardiac failure; JVP, jugular venous pressure.)

Diagram labels:

JVP — elevated in CCF

BP — take when patient is relaxed; check cuff size is correct

pulses — check radial, femoral, popliteal, and foot pulses; look for weak pulses (peripheral vascular disease); radiofemoral delay; atrial fibrillation; bruits (generalized atherosclerosis)

urine — blood or protein (renal disease)

oedema — peripheral oedema (CCF)

eyes — hypertensive retinopathy; diabetic retinal eye disease

heart — displaced apex (left ventricular hypertrophy or dilatation); harsh murmur (coarctation; if this is suspected, listen for a murmur over the scapula due to collaterals)

abdomen — hepatomegaly and ascites (cardiac failure); bruits over renal arteries (renal artery stenosis); abdominal aortic aneurysm (generalized atherosclerosis); palpable kidneys (polycystic kidney disease)

peripheries — cold (peripheral vascular disease)

Investigations for hypertension
blood tests—renal function and electrolytes, blood lipid profile, blood glucose
ECG—may provide evidence of LVH (i.e. R wave in V5 >25 mm, deep S wave in V2 or R wave in V5 added to S wave in V2 greater than 50 mm, R wave in AVL >11 mm, lateral T wave inversion)
echocardiogram—LVH, usually concentric in nature (i.e. left ventricular wall thickness >1.1 cm); performed routinely at some centres because LVH is thought to be a valuable indicator of prognosis

Fig. 24.3 Investigations for hypertension. (LVH, left ventricular hypertrophy.)

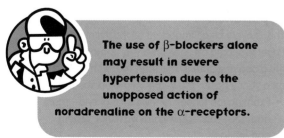

The use of β-blockers alone may result in severe hypertension due to the unopposed action of noradrenaline on the α-receptors.

Investigation of secondary hypertension

All patients should have the investigations listed in Fig. 24.3. For those patients at high risk of secondary hypertension the following screening tests should exclude most causative conditions:

- 24-hour urine protein and creatinine clearance to exclude marked renal pathology.
- 24-hour urine catecholamines or vanillylmandelic acid (VMA) and 5-hydroxy indole acetic acid (5HIAA) to exclude phaeochromocytoma and carcinoid syndrome, respectively. (Three sets of urinary catecholamines should be tested.)
- 24-hour urine cortisol excretion and dexamethasone suppression test to exclude Cushing's syndrome.
- Renal ultrasound—to reveal any overt structural abnormality (e.g. phaeochromocytoma, small kidney, or polycystic kidneys.
- Renal perfusion scan (diethylenetriamine pentaacetic acid, DTPA) with and without angiotensin-converting enzyme (ACE) inhibition to exclude renal artery stenosis. The kidney in renal artery stenosis depends heavily upon increased levels of angiotensin II to provide adequate blood pressure for renal perfusion. This is abruptly stopped by the administration of an

ACE inhibitor and the reduction in renal blood flow that results can be detected by the scan. If this test is positive then renal angiography is the gold standard investigation to confirm the diagnosis.

MANAGEMENT OF HYPERTENSION

Importance of treating hypertension

Hypertension is a common disorder that if left untreated damages a number of systems. Complications of hypertension include:

- Cardiac failure.
- Renal failure.
- Stroke.
- Ischaemic heart disease.
- Peripheral vascular disease.

This end-organ damage can largely be prevented by adequate blood pressure control.

Hypertension is, however, difficult to diagnose because patients are often asymptomatic; treatment is therefore difficult because patients are less likely to comply with drug regimens or follow-up visits to their doctor.

Non-pharmacological management

This is important because in patients who have mild hypertension it may result in a moderate decrease in blood pressure of 11/8 mmHg and this may be sufficient to avoid the need for drug therapy. The following non-pharmacological treatments are recognized:

- Weight loss.
- Reduction in alcohol consumption—the maximum recommended weekly intakes are 21 units for men and 14 units for women.
- Reduction in salt intake.
- Regular exercise.

All other risk factors for ischaemic heart disease should be sought and treated in these patients as a matter of routine.

Pharmacological management

There are many effective agents (Fig. 24.4). The main categories are as follows:

- Diuretics.
- Antiadrenergic agents—β-blockers (β-adrenoceptor antagonists), α-blockers (α-adrenoceptor antagonists), and centrally acting agents.
- Calcium channel blockers.
- Angiotensin-converting enzyme inhibitors and angiotensin II receptor blockers.
- Vasodilators.

These agents may be used alone or in combination to achieve good blood pressure control. Remember that patient compliance is likely to be better if:

- The disease and its complications have been fully explained.
- The treatment options have been discussed with the patient.
- The drugs used have been explained and common side effects discussed.
- Once-daily preparations are used.
- Polypharmacy is avoided (i.e. the drug regimen is kept as simple as possible by using a higher dose of a single agent before adding another drug).

Recommended treatment of hypertension

The 1997 British Hypertension Society guidelines for the treatment of hypertension suggest that:

- Observation and non-pharmacological treatment are appropriate for patients under 60 years of age who have no end-organ damage and a diastolic blood pressure of 90–99 mmHg.
- Drug treatment is indicated for older patients (over 60 years of age) who have a systolic blood pressure over 160 mmHg even if the diastolic is less than 90 mmHg because isolated systolic hypertension is an independent risk factor for stroke.
- Non-pharmacological measures should be instituted for all patients.

These guidelines are constantly changing and clinical practice varies from hospital to hospital.

Follow-up of patients who have hypertension

This is every bit as important as the initial treatment. Patients should be seen on a 1- or 2-monthly basis until the blood pressure is less than 140/90 mmHg and then on a yearly basis. The yearly follow-up should involve:

- Examination to look for evidence of end-organ damage—especially cardiovascular system and retinas.

Drugs used to treat hypertension				
Class of drug	**Examples**	**Indications**	**Contraindications**	**Adverse effects**
diuretics	thiazides (e.g. bendrofluazide), loop diuretics (e.g. frusemide)	mild hypertension or in conjunction with other agents for more severe hypertension	thiazides exacerbate diabetes mellitus; all diuretics should be avoided in patients who have gout if possible	hypokalaemia, dehydration, exacerbation of renal impairment, gout
anti-adrenergic agents	β-blockers (e.g. atenolol, propanolol, metoprolol)	moderate to severe hypertension (note that they are antianginal)	asthma, cardiac failure, severe peripheral vascular disease	postural hypotension, bronchospasm, fatigue, impotence, cold extremities
	α-blockers (e.g. prazosin, doxazosin)	moderate to severe hypertension	postural hypotension	
	centrally acting agents (e.g. methyldopa)	moderate hypertension (safe during pregnancy)	postural hypotension, galactorrhoea, gynaecomastia, haemolytic anaemia	
calcium channel blockers	nifedipine, amlodipine,	moderate hypertension*	cardiac failure, heart block (2nd or 3rd degree)—these are contraindications for mainly verapamil and diltiazem	postural hypotension, headache, flushing, ankle oedema
ACE inhibitors	captopril, enalapril, lisinopril	moderate to severe hypertension, especially with cardiac failure	renal artery stenosis, pregnancy	postural hypotension, dry cough, loss of taste, renal failure, hyperkalaemia
angiotensin-II receptor blockers	losartan, valsartan	moderate to severe hypertension, especially with cardiac failure	renal artery stenosis, pregnancy	postural hypotension, renal failure, hyperkalaemia
vasodilators	hydralazine	moderate to severe hypertension	SLE	postural hypotension, headache, lupus-like syndrome
	sodium nitroprusside (as an intravenous infusion)	malignant hypertension	weakness, cyanide toxicity if drug not protected from light	

Fig. 24.4 Overview of drugs used to treat hypertension. (ACE, angiotensin-converting enzyme; SLE, systemic lupus erythematosus; *diltiazem and verapamil are less commonly used for hypertension because they have a more pronounced action on heart muscle and conductive tissue, respectively; diltiazem is used predominantly for angina and verapamil for its antiarrhythmic affects.)

- ECG.
- Blood tests for urea, creatinine, and electrolytes—these may be deranged due to renal damage secondary to hypertension or to the drug therapy or both.
- Echocardiography if the patient had left ventricular hypertrophy at diagnosis—it is appropriate to repeat the echocardiography until the hypertrophy has resolved.
- A screen of risk factors for ischaemic heart disease (i.e. blood lipid profile and blood glucose) and lifestyle advice if necessary.

PHAEOCHROMOCYTOMA

Phaeochromocytoma is a tumour of the chromaffin cells—90% occur within the adrenal medulla and 10% are extramedullary; 10% are malignant.

Clinical features
Paroxysmal catecholamine secretion results in a variety of signs and symptoms including:
- Hypertension.
- Headaches.

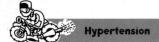

- Sweating attacks.
- Postural hypotension.
- Acute pulmonary oedema.

These symptoms are characteristically paroxysmal, but patients may have persistent hypertension.

Investigations

Investigations include:

- ECG—ST elevation or T wave inversion may be seen transiently.
- Echocardiography—shows left ventricular hypertrophy or dilated cardiomyopathy.
- 24-hour urinary catecholamines or VMA—these are raised. (At least three measurements should be taken due to the intermittent nature of the catecholamine excretion.)

- Computed tomography scan of the adrenals or meta-iodobenzylguanidine (MIBG) scan if the tumour is extra-adrenal.
- Selective venous sampling.

Management

Careful blood pressure control is vital before any invasive procedure as follows:

- Initially α-blocker is used (phenoxybenzamine an irreversible α-blocker is commonly used).
- β-Blockade may then be added if required—the use of β–blockers alone may result in severe hypertension due to the unopposed action of noradrenaline on the α-receptors.

The tumour is then removed surgically.

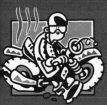

25. Congenital Heart Disease

DEFINITION OF CONGENITAL HEART DISEASE

Congenital heart disease refers to cardiac lesions present from birth.

CAUSES OF CONGENITAL HEART DISEASE

Many factors both genetic and environmental affect cardiac development in the uterus; therefore not surprisingly, no one cause can explain all cases (Fig. 25.1). These include:

- Maternal rubella—in addition to cataracts, deafness, and microcephaly, this can cause patent ductus arteriosus (PDA) and pulmonary stenosis.
- Fetal alcohol syndrome—associated with cardiac defects (as well as microcephaly, micrognathia, microphthalmia, and growth retardation).
- Maternal systemic lupus erythematosus—associated with fetal complete heart block (due to transplacental passage of anti-Ro antibodies).

There are many genetic associations with congenital heart disease, including:

- Trisomy 21—endocardial cushion defects, atrial septal defect (ASD), ventricular septal defect (VSD), Fallot's tetralogy.

Cardiac malformations
ventricular septal defect (VSD)
atrial septal defect (ASD)
patent ductus arteriosus (PDA)
pulmonary stenosis—causes cyanosis if severe
coarctation of the aorta
aortic stenosis
Fallot's tetralogy—causes cyanosis
transposition of the great arteries—causes cyanosis
other causes of cyanotic congenital heart disease—pulmonary atresia, hypoplastic left heart, severe Ebstein's anomaly with ASD

Fig. 25.1 Cardiac malformations (in descending order of incidence).

- Turner's syndrome (XO)—coarctation of the aorta.
- Marfan syndrome—aortic dilatation and aortic and mitral regurgitation.
- Kartagener's syndrome—dextrocardia.

COMPLICATIONS OF CONGENITAL HEART DISEASE

Before discussing individual lesions it is important to have a grasp of the significance of congenital heart disease. Lesions have effects depending upon their size and location. These include:

- Cyanosis—defined as the presence of more than 5 g/dL of reduced haemoglobin in arterial blood. Central cyanosis can be caused by congenital heart disease due to shunting of venous blood straight into the arterial circulation bypassing the lungs. This type of cyanosis does not therefore respond to increasing the concentration of inspired oxygen.
- Congestive cardiac failure—this occurs due to the inability of the heart to maintain sufficient tissue perfusion as a result of the cardiac lesion. This may occur in infancy (e.g. due to a large VSD or transposition of the great arteries), or in adulthood in less severe conditions.
- Pulmonary hypertension—this occurs as a result of an abnormal increase in pulmonary blood flow due to a left-to-right shunt (e.g. ASD, VSD, PDA). This increased flow results in changes to the pulmonary vessels with smooth muscle hypertrophy and obliterative changes. The pulmonary vascular resistance increases causing pulmonary hypertension. Eventually pulmonary pressure exceeds systemic pressure causing reversal of the shunt and this results in a syndrome of cyanotic heart disease called Eisenmenger's syndrome.
- Infective endocarditis—congenital heart disease may result in lesions prone to bacterial colonization. Appropriate antibiotic prophylaxis should be taken to prevent this.
- Sudden death—this may be due to arrhythmias (more common in these disorders) or outflow tract obstruction as seen in aortic stenosis.

Notes on cyanosis:
Central cyanosis is cyanosis of the tongue and lips.
Peripheral cyanosis is cyanosis of the peripheries (feet, hands, etc)
Cyanosis caused by pulmonary disease or cardiac failure improves on increasing inspired oxygen.
Cyanosis caused by a right to left shunt bypassing the lungs does not improve on increasing inspired oxygen.

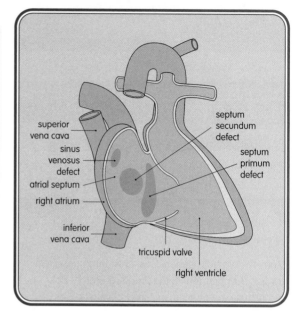

Fig. 25.2 Location of the three main types of atrial septal defect: here the heart is viewed from the right side. The right atrial and ventricular walls have been omitted to reveal the septum.

ATRIAL SEPTAL DEFECT

Although a common cause of congenital heart disease this disorder is often not diagnosed early because it is often clinically difficult to detect.

There are three main types of ASD based on the location of the defect in the atrial septum (Fig. 25.2):

- Septum primum (also called ostium primum ASD) —this defect lies adjacent to the atrioventricular valves and these are often also abnormal and incompetent.
- Septum secundum (also called ostium secundum ASD)—the most common form of ASD, it is mid-septal in location.
- Sinus venosus ASD—this lies high in the septum and may be associated with anomalous pulmonary venous drainage (where one of the pulmonary veins drains into the right atrium instead of the left).

Clinical features

The magnitude of the left-to-right shunt depends upon the size of the defect and also the relative pressures on the left and right sides of the heart.

History

In early life patients are usually asymptomatic. In adult life, however, symptoms of dyspnoea, fatigue, and recurrent chest infections occur.

As time goes by the increased pulmonary blood flow results in pulmonary hypertension and eventually reversal of the shunt and Eisenmenger's syndrome.

On examination

The findings on examination of a patient who has an ASD (Fig. 25.3) depend upon the following factors:

- Size of the ASD.
- Presence or absence of pulmonary hypertension.
- Presence of shunt reversal.

The second heart sound is widely split because closure of the pulmonary valve is delayed due to increased pulmonary blood flow. The splitting is fixed in relation to respiration because the communication between the atria prevents the normal pressure differential between right and left sides that occurs during respiration. This is referred to as fixed splitting of the second heart sound.

The increased pulmonary blood flow causes a mid-systolic pulmonary flow murmur.

If pulmonary hypertension has developed, there is reduction of the left-to-right shunt and the pulmonary flow murmur disappears; instead there is a loud pulmonary component to the second heart sound because the increased pressure causes the pulmonary valve to slam shut.

If Eisenmenger's syndrome occurs the patient becomes centrally cyanosed and develops finger clubbing.

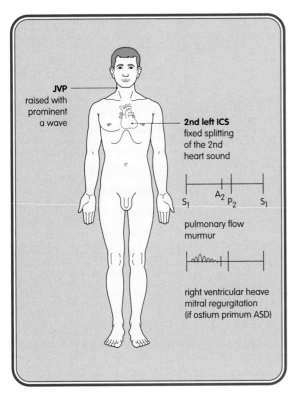

Fig. 25.3 Physical findings in all patients who have an atrial septal defect (ASD). If the ASD is large and there is pulmonary hypertension check for loud P_2 at the second left intercostal space (ICS) and a prominent right ventricular heave. If there is shunt reversal you will find clubbing, central cyanosis, and signs of congestive cardiac failure (i.e. peripheral oedema, ascites and bilateral basal crepitations). (A_2, aortic component of second heart sound; JVP, jugular venous pressure; S_1, first heart sound.)

Eisenmenger's syndrome can occur in any condition involving a left to right shunt. With worsening pulmonary hypertension the shunt eventually reverses (changes to right to left) causing blood to bypass the lungs and resulting in profound cyanosis that is not responsive to oxygen therapy. There is no treatment at this late stage.

Investigation
Electrocardiography
Patients who have ostium secundum ASD usually have right axis deviation. Those who have an ostium primum defect have left axis deviation.

Chest radiography
The pulmonary artery appears dilated and its branches are prominent. The enlarged right atrium can be seen at the right heart border and the enlarged right ventricle causes rounding of the left heart border.

Echocardiography
The right side of the heart is dilated and the pulmonary artery is dilated. The ASD may be directly visualized and a jet of blood may be seen passing through it. Associated mitral or tricuspid valve incompetence may be seen.

Cardiac catheterization
This again reveals the ASD because the catheter can be passed across it. Serial oxygen saturation measurements are made at different levels from the superior vena cava through the atrium and the right ventricle into the pulmonary artery. At the level of the left-to-right shunt there will be a step up increase of the oxygen saturation as blood from the left side enters the right. This measurement can be used to calculate the size of the shunt, which helps decide on whether operative correction of the ASD is required.

Management
If there are signs of congestive cardiac failure, diuretics and angiotensin-converting enzyme inhibitors may be of benefit.

An ASD carries a risk of infective endocarditis so the appropriate prophylactic measures should be taken.

The primary aim in these patients is to diagnose the ASD early and evaluate its severity to be able to repair the defect before pulmonary hypertension occurs. Once the patient has developed pulmonary hypertension repair does not stop its deterioration.

All ASDs with pulmonary to systemic flow ratios exceeding 1.5:1 should be repaired.

Operative closure requires cardiopulmonary bypass and involves a median sternotomy scar.

A new technique has been developed where the ASD is closed using a clam-shell shaped device that can be introduced via a cardiac catheter and involves only an arterial and a venous puncture.

When asked about the management of any valve disease or congenital defect many students forget that antibiotic prophylaxis is probably one of the most important aspects of management—so don't forget to put it high on your list of priorities.

VENTRICULAR SEPTAL DEFECT

This is the most common congenital cardiac abnormality. The ventricular septum is made up of two main components:

- The membranous septum—situated high in the septum and relatively small. This is the most common site for a VSD.
- The muscular septum—this is lower and defects here may be multiple.

Clinical features
History
In the neonate a small VSD will be asymptomatic, but a large VSD will result in the development of left ventricular failure. This occurs because in the neonate pulmonary pressures are very high (because they are in utero) and a right-to-left shunt occurs via the VSD; if this is very large the left ventricle cannot cope and fails. The signs of LVF in a neonate are as follows:

- Failure to thrive, feeding difficulties, and sweating on feeding.
- Tachypnoea and intercostal recession.
- Hepatomegaly.

The adult who has a VSD may be asymptomatic or may present with dyspnoea due to pulmonary hypertension, (which develops as a consequence of the left-to-right shunt) or Eisenmenger's syndrome.

Examination
The findings on examination of a patient who has a VSD (Fig. 25.4) vary according to the following criteria:

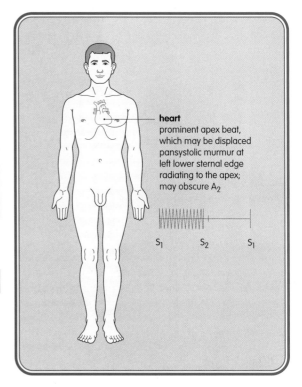

heart
prominent apex beat, which may be displaced pansystolic murmur at left lower sternal edge radiating to the apex; may obscure A_2

S_1　　S_2　　S_1

Fig. 25.4 Physical findings in all patients who have a ventricular septal defect (VSD). If the VSD is large the apex is displaced and pulmonary hypertension may develop resulting in a loud P_2 and right ventricular heave. Eisenmenger's syndrome may also develop with clubbing and cyanosis and disappearance of the pansystolic murmur. (A_2, aortic component of second heart sound.)

- Size of the VSD—a small VSD causes a loud pansystolic murmur that radiates to the apex and axilla. A very large VSD causes a less loud pansystolic murmur, but may be associated with signs of left ventricular and right ventricular hypertrophy.
- Presence or absence of pulmonary hypertension.
- Presence of shunt reversal.

Investigation
Chest radiography
This may show an enlarged left ventricle with prominent pulmonary vascular markings. Pulmonary oedema may be seen in infants.

Echocardiography
This will show the VSD and its size and location.

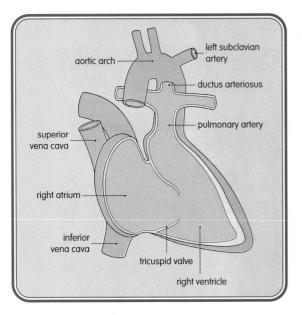

Fig. 25.5 Position of the ductus arteriosus.

Management

Approximately 30% of cases close spontaneously, most of these by the time the child is 3 years of age. Some do not close until the child is 10 years old. Defects near the valve ring or near the outlet of the ventricle do not usually close.

Operative closure is the treatment of choice and is recommended for all lesions that have not undergone spontaneous closure. Some small lesions are left; such a patient may be a case in finals and has a loud pansystolic murmur.

A VSD is a risk factor for infective endocarditis so the appropriate prophylactic measures should be taken.

PATENT DUCTUS ARTERIOSUS

In the fetus most of the output of the right ventricle bypasses the lungs via the ductus arteriosus. This vessel joins the pulmonary trunk (artery) to the descending aorta distal to the left subclavian artery (Fig. 25.5). The ductus arteriosus normally closes about 1 month after birth in full-term infants and takes longer to close in premature infants.

Clinical features

The factors that determine the nature of the clinical features are the same as in VSD and ASD (i.e. the size

of the defect, the presence of pulmonary hypertension, and the development of Eisenmenger's syndrome).

A patent PDA is more likely in babies born at high altitude, probably due to the low atmospheric oxygen concentration. This lesion is also common in babies who have fetal rubella syndrome.

History

A small PDA is asymptomatic, but a large defect causes a large left-to-right shunt and may lead to left ventricular failure with pulmonary oedema causing failure to thrive and tachypnoea.

Adults who have undiagnosed PDA may develop pulmonary hypertension and present with dyspnoea.

Differential cyanosis occurs in adults with reversal of the shunt as the venous blood enters the systemic circulation below the subclavian arteries causing cyanosis of the lower extremities whereas the arms remain pink.

On examination

The classical findings in a patient who has PDA (Fig. 25.6) are:
- Collapsing high-volume pulses—this is due to the effect of the run-off of blood back down the ductus.
- A loud continuous machinery murmur heard in the second left intercostal space.
- A palpable thrill in the same place.

Management

The management of PDA involves two stages:
- Pharmacological closure in neonates—indomethacin may induce closure if given early.
- Operative closure of the PDA—this can be performed as an open procedure where the PDA is ligated or divided. Alternatively a percutaneous approach can be performed with introduction of an occluding device via a cardiac catheter. Antibiotic prophylaxis is required for all patients before operative correction because PDA is a risk factor for infective endocarditis.

COARCTATION OF THE AORTA

In this condition there is a congenital narrowing of the aorta, usually beyond the left subclavian artery.

There are two main types:
- Infantile type—this presents soon after birth with heart failure.

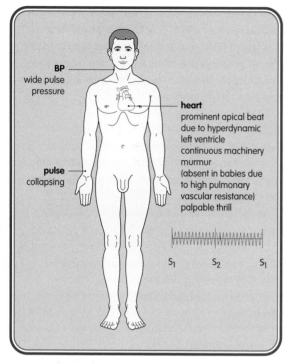

Fig. 25.6 Physical findings in all patients who have patent ductus arteriosus (PDA). In patients who have a large PDA there is a loud pulmonary component of the second heart sound (P_2) due to pulmonary hypertension and the murmur is soft or absent. In those who have Eisenmenger's syndrome there is differential cyanosis and the toes are clubbed.

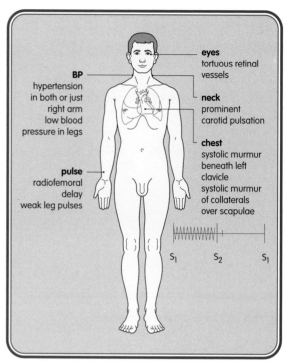

Fig. 25.7 Physical findings in patients who have coarctation of the aorta. If the coarctation is severe there is a continuous murmur beneath the left clavicle and there are signs of left ventricular failure (bilateral basal crepitations and audible third heart sound.)

- Adult type—the obstruction develops more gradually and presents in early adulthood. This type is associated with a high incidence of bicuspid aortic valve.

An adaptive response to the coarctation develops in those patients who do not present in infancy. This involves the development of collateral blood vessels, which divert blood from the proximal aorta to other peripheral arteries bypassing the obstruction. These collaterals are seen around the scapula as tortuous vessels that can sometimes be palpated and as prominent posterior intercostal arteries that cause rib notching visible on a chest radiography. These collaterals take some years to develop and are rarely seen before 6 years of age.

Clinical features
History
Infants may present with failure to thrive and tachypnoea secondary to left ventricular failure.

Alternatively coarctation may present as rapid severe cardiac failure with the infant in extremis.

Adults whose condition is not diagnosed in childhood may present with:
- Hypertension diagnosed at routine medical testing.
- Symptoms of leg claudication.
- Left ventricular failure.
- Subarachnoid haemorrhage from associated berry aneurysm.
- Angina pectoris due to premature heart disease.

On examination
Careful examination of these patients is vital because the diagnosis must not be missed. The physical findings in patients who have coarctation of the aorta are shown in Fig. 25.7. Check for:
- Blood pressure—it is always important to take blood pressure in both arms whenever performing the cardiovascular examination. Aortic dissection and coarctation where the obstruction is proximal to the

left subclavian artery both cause a pressure differential between the arms. The blood pressure in the legs is also lower than in the arms.

- Radiofemoral delay and weak leg pulses—it is important to always look for radiofemoral delay because it is diagnostic of this condition.
- A heaving displaced apex beat due to left ventricular hypertrophy.
- Murmurs—the coarctation may cause a systolic murmur (or a continuous murmur if the narrowing is very tight). This is located below the left clavicle. The collaterals around the scapulas cause an ejection systolic murmur that can be heard over the scapulas. There may be a murmur associated with a bicuspid aortic valve, which is ejection systolic in nature and is located over the aortic area.

Investigation
Electrocardiography
This reveals left ventricular hypertrophy and often right bundle branch block.

Chest radiography
Rib notching may be seen in children over 6 years of age. (Because the first and second intercostal arteries arise from the vertebral arteries there is no rib notching on these ribs.) The aortic knuckle is absent and a double knuckle is seen (made up of the dilated subclavian artery above and the poststenotic dilatation of the aorta below).

Echocardiography
The coarctation can be visualized as can any associated lesion. Coarctation is associated with a number of other congenital abnormalities (e.g. transposition of the great arteries, septum primum ASD, mitral valve disease, bicuspid aortic valve).

Cardiac catheterization
This localizes the coarctation accurately and also provides more information on associated lesions.

Management
The most popular first-line treatment is an operation to relieve the obstruction. Without correction the prognosis is extremely poor and most patients die by 40 years of age.

Balloon angioplasty is another option, but this is usually reserved for the treatment of postsurgical restenosis.

Coarctation may be complicated by infective endocarditis so antibiotic prophylaxis should be used.

OTHER CAUSES OF CONGENITAL HEART DISEASE

The conditions discussed above are those most likely to be seen in the examination situation. There are, however, a number of less common congenital cardiac abnormalities and these are discussed in Fig. 25.8.

NOTES ON PULMONARY HYPERTENSION AND EISENMENGER'S SYNDROME

Pulmonary hypertension
This causes mild dyspnoea when the shunt is from left to right and severe dyspnoea on shunt reversal.

Signs on examination include:
- Dominant a wave in the jugular venous pulse.
- Palpable and loud pulmonary component of second heart sound.
- Ejection systolic murmur in pulmonary area due to increased flow.
- Right ventricular heave.
- Tricuspid regurgitation if the right ventricle dilates.

The investigation of choice is echocardiography, which allows assessment of the pulmonary pressures. This is vital because an operation should be performed before significant pulmonary hypertension develops.

Eisenmenger's syndrome
This refers to the situation where a congenital cardiac abnormality initially causes acyanotic heart disease, but cyanotic heart disease develops as a consequence of raised pulmonary pressure and shunt reversal.

These clinical features are also seen in patients who have cyanotic congenital heart disease (i.e. where the lesion results in a right-to-left shunt from the outset). Cyanosis develops when the level of reduced haemoglobin is over 5 g/dL.

Dyspnoea is usually relatively mild considering the profound hypoxia these patients have (oxygen saturations of 50% are not uncommon).

Uncommon causes of congenital cardiac abnormalities			
Congenital cardiac defect	**Anatomical abnormality**	**Clinical features**	**Treatment**
congenital aortic stenosis (acyanotic)	stenosis may be valvular (most common), subvalvular, or supravalvular; note Williams syndrome—autosomal dominant condition with hypercalcaemia and supravalvular aortic stenosis	more common in males; child may be hypotensive, dyspnoeic, and sweaty; increased incidence of angina and sudden death, especially on exertion; ejection systolic murmur heard in the 2nd right ICS; may be signs of left ventricular strain (heaving apex) and failure (S_3, tachycardia, and bilateral basal crackles)	operative correction of the stenosis is the treatment of choice; in very small infants valvuloplasty is preferred in the first instance
hypoplastic left heart (cyanotic)	underdevelopment of all or part of the left side of the heart	heart failure occurs in the 1st week of life; echocardiography is diagnostic	surgical treatment is the only option and the mortality rate is extremely high
pulmonary artery stenosis (cyanotic only if severe)	stenosis at one or many points along the pulmonary arteries; associated with Fallot's tetralogy in some cases; complication of maternal rubella infection	if mild the patient may be asymptomatic with signs of RVH (i.e. left parasternal heave) and a pulmonary ejection systolic murmur; if severe blood flows from the right side to the left through the foramen ovale and the child is cyanosed and dyspnoeic	diagnosis is confirmed by echocardiography; pulmonary angioplasty may provide a definitive cure; if there is a recurrence or the lesion is not suitable for pulmonary angioplasty the obstruction may be removed surgically
tetralogy of Fallot (cyanotic)	four components—1. VSD; 2. pulmonary stenosis; 3. over-riding aorta; 4. RVH—blood flow therefore passes from the right ventricle through the VSD and through the aorta, resulting in a right to left shunt	most children present with cyanosis within the 1st year of life; patients may have 'spells' of intense cyanosis from time to time due to a sudden increase in the right to left shunt—these attacks may be terminated by squatting, which increases systemic resistance and therefore reduces the right to left shunt	total surgical correction is the treatment of first choice; in very young infants who have severe pulmonary atresia a palliative operation to reduce the pulmonary obstruction usually provides relief and a definitive procedure can be carried out later when the risk is lower
complete transposition of the great arteries (cyanotic)	the aorta arises from the right ventricle and the pulmonary artery arises from the left ventricle—the two circulations are therefore parallel; death is rapid if there is no communication between them so it is common to see an ASD, VSD, or PDA as well in these infants	early cardiac failure and cyanosis are the most common presenting features; symptoms are less severe in those infants who have a large communication between the two sides; diagnosis is made by echocardiography and cardiac catheterization	medical treatment of cardiac failure and the use of prostaglandin E_1 to prevent postnatal closure of the ductus may help; operative procedures to create a large ASD may also help in the short term; surgical correction of the transposition is the definitive treatment

Fig. 25.8 Uncommon causes of congenital cardiac abnormalities. (ASD, atrial septal defect; ICS, intercostal space; PDA, patent ductus arteriosus; RVH, right ventricular hypertrophy; S_3, third heart sound, VSD, ventricular septal defect.)

Complications include:
- Clubbing—develops in the fingers and toes.
- Polycythaemia and hyperviscosity—with resulting complications of stroke and venous thrombosis. Regular venesection is the treatment of choice.
- Cerebral abscesses—especially in children.
- Paradoxical emboli—emboli from venous thrombosis may pass across the shunt and give rise to systemic infarcts.

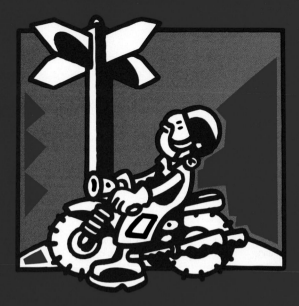

SELF-ASSESSMENT

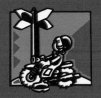
Indicate whether each answer is true or false.

1. **The following are signs of right ventricular failure:**

a) Hypotension.
b) Hepatomegaly.
c) Raised jugular venous pressure.
d) Bilateral basal crepitations.
e) Mid-diastolic murmur.

2. **The following chest radiograph signs suggest left ventricular failure:**

a) Cardiomegaly.
b) Upper lobe blood diversion.
c) Pleural effusion.
d) Oligaemic lung fields.
e) Kerley B lines.

3. **The following are contraindications for the use of β-blockers (β-adrenoceptor antagonists):**

a) Cardiac failure.
b) Asthma.
c) Peripheral vascular disease.
d) Diabetes mellitus.
e) Hypotension, blood pressure less than 90/60 mmHg.

4. **The differential diagnosis for chest pain includes:**

a) Myocardial infarction.
b) Oesophagitis.
c) Pulmonary embolus.
d) Cholecystitis.
e) Aortic dissection.

5. **Dissection of the thoracic aorta may give the following:**

a) Hypotension.
b) ST elevation on the ECG.
c) Raised jugular venous pressure.
d) Hemiplegia.
e) A loud murmur radiating from the apex to the axilla.

6. **The following are causes of acute life-threatening dyspnoea:**

a) Myocardial infarction.
b) Pulmonary embolus.
c) Pneumothorax.
d) Ventricular or supraventricular tachyarrhythmia.
e) Bacterial endocarditis.

7. **The following are clinical signs found in infective endocarditis:**

a) Clubbing.
b) Haematuria.
c) Pyrexia.
d) Rashes.
e) Focal neurological defect.

8. **The following are risk factors for ischaemic heart disease:**

a) Hypertension.
b) Moderate alcohol intake.
c) Female sex.
d) Hypercholesterolaemia.
e) Increasing age.

9. **The following may exacerbate angina:**

a) Sleep.
b) Tachyarrhythmia.
c) Anaemia.
d) High altitude.
e) Cold air.

10. **The following are classical features of cardiac syncope:**

a) Gradual onset.
b) Warning symptoms.
c) Rapid recovery.
d) Residual neurological deficit.
e) Precipitated by sudden turning of the head.

11. **The following manoeuvres cause vagal stimulation:**

a) Straining against a closed glottis.
b) Carotid sinus massage.
c) Immersing face in cold water.
d) Pleasurable stimuli.
e) Micturition.

12. **The following are causes of a pansystolic murmur:**

a) Mitral regurgitation.
b) Aortic regurgitation.
c) Tricuspid regurgitation.
d) Atrial septal defect.
e) Aortic stenosis.

199

13. The following are true of mitral regurgitation:

a) A mid-diastolic sound may be heard.
b) It may occur suddenly post myocardial infarction.
c) The apex is often displaced.
d) Atrial fibrillation may be a complicating factor.
e) Chest radiography is the best diagnostic test.

14. The following conditions require antibiotic prophylaxis before dental procedures:

a) Prosthetic aortic valve.
b) Ventricular septal defect.
c) Floppy mitral valve with coexistent mitral regurgitation.
d) Enlarged left ventricle.
e) A history of infective endocarditis in the past.

15. The following are complications of hypertension:

a) Renal failure.
b) Cardiac failure.
c) Diabetes mellitus.
d) Cerebrovascular event.
e) Ischaemic heart disease.

16. The following should be considered as possible signs of a positive exercise test:

a) ST segment depression.
b) Exercise-induced hypotension.
c) Exercise-induced ventricular tachycardia.
d) Lack of adequate tachycardic response to exercise.
e) Leg pain at peak exercise.

17. The following are recognized causes of atrial fibrillation:

a) Ischaemic heart disease.
b) Hyperthyroidism.
c) Pulmonary embolus.
d) Jaundice.
e) Septicaemia.

18. The following are indications for anticoagulating a patient who has atrial fibrillation with warfarin:

a) Age under 60 years.
b) Associated mitral stenosis.
c) Atrial fibrillation of more than 24 hours' duration.
d) A history of cerebral thromboembolism.
e) Associated left ventricular failure.

19. The following statements are true of adenosine:

a) It blocks conduction throughout the sinoatrial node.
b) It has a half life of approx 8–10 s.
c) It is contraindicated in asthma.
d) It may cause slowing of the ventricular rate in atrial flutter.
e) It will cause slowing of the ventricular rate in ventricular tachycardia.

20. The following are true of ventricular tachycardia:

a) It is a life-threatening condition.
b) It may be caused by myocardial ischaemia.
c) It may be caused by hypokalaemia.
d) Amiodarone may be used to prevent recurrent episodes of ventricular tachycardia.
e) Acute ongoing ventricular tachycardia should be treated initially with drugs.

21. The following are true of digoxin:

a) It acts to slow conduction through the atrioventricular node.
b) It is contraindicated in Wolff–Parkinson–White syndrome.
c) It may cardiovert a re-entry supraventricular tachycardia to sinus rhythm.
d) Its main route of excretion is the liver.
e) It has a very short half-life.

22. The following are signs of coarctation of the aorta:

a) Radiofemoral delay in the pulses.
b) Rib notching.
c) Bruits heard over the scapula.
d) Ankle oedema.
e) Atrial fibrillation.

23. The following statements about infective endocarditis are true:

a) The most common causative organisms in Western countries are the *Streptococcus viridans* group.
b) Fungal infections are commonly seen on the aortic valve.
c) *Staphylococcus aureus* is associated with a benign slowly progressive disease.
d) Enterococci are very rare.
e) Gram-negative bacteria and diphtheroids are encountered soon after valve operations.

24. Functions of the recovery position include:

a) To prevent the tongue from obstructing the airway.
b) To prevent neck injury.
c) To minimize the risk of aspiration of gastric contents.
d) To maintain a straight airway.
e) To enable cardiopulmonary resuscitation to be carried out.

25. Complications of prosthetic heart valves are as follows:

a) Thromboembolic events.
b) Dehiscence of the valve ring.
c) Increased risk of infective endocarditis.
d) Failure of the valve 5 years after placement.
e) Need for anticoagulation in patients who have porcine valves.

26. The following statements are true of thiazide diuretics:

a) They act at the level of the distal convoluted tubule.
b) They may cause gout.
c) Diabetic control may deteriorate.
d) Hypokalaemia may occur.
e) They cause ototoxicity.

27. The following drugs have been shown to reduce the mortality rate for patients who have cardiac failure:

a) Diuretics.
b) Angiotensin-converting enzyme inhibitors.
c) Nitrates and hydralazine used in combination.
d) Metolozone.
e) β-Blockers (β-adrenoceptor antagonists).

28. The following are classified as high-output states:

a) Hypertension .
b) Sepsis.
c) Hypothyroidism.
d) Pregnancy.
e) Arteriovenous malformations.

29. The following are examples of cyanotic congenital cardiac disease:

a) Ventricular septal defect.
b) Patent ductus arteriosus.
c) Tetralogy of Fallot.
d) Congenital aortic stenosis.
e) Transposition of the great arteries.

30. Cardiac causes of clubbing are as follows:

a) Uncomplicated atrial septal defect.
b) Chronic infective endocarditis.
c) Atrial fibrillation.
d) Acute endocarditis.
e) Empyema.

31. Characteristic features of the jugular venous pulse are as follows:

a) It has a single pulsation.
b) The v wave coincides with ventricular systole.
c) It falls if the patient becomes more upright.
d) It cannot be obliterated.
e) There is no a wave in atrial fibrillation.

32. The following statements are true of the apex beat:

a) It is the lowest and most lateral point at which the cardiac impulse can be felt.
b) It is displaced downwards and laterally if the left ventricle is enlarged.
c) It is thrusting in mitral stenosis.
d) It is thrusting in aortic regurgitation.
e) It is heaving in aortic stenosis.

33. The following lipid lowering drugs have been shown to reduce cardiovascular mortality rates:

a) Cholestyramine.
b) Simvastatin.
c) Gemfibrozil.
d) Nicotinic acid.
e) Cerivastatin.

34. The following leads represent the inferior myocardium:

a) I, AVL, and V6.
b) V2, V3, and V4.
c) AVR and V1.
d) V1–V6.
e) II, III, and AVF.

35. After a myocardial infarction a patient should if possible be discharged on the following drugs:

a) A statin.
b) Aspirin.
c) A calcium channel blocker.
d) An angiotensin-converting enzyme inhibitor.
e) A β-blocker (β-adrenoceptor antagonist).

36. The following are possible causes of electromechanical dissociation:

a) Pulmonary embolus.
b) Tension pneumothorax.
c) Hypertension.
d) Dehydration.
e) Hypocalcaemia.

37. The following are true of hypertrophic obstructive cardiomyopathy:

a) The heart is always enlarged.
b) Patients may present with dyspnoea and/or syncope.
c) There may be a systolic murmur on auscultation.
d) The disease is genetically acquired.
e) Echocardiography is often diagnostic.

38. Mitral stenosis has the following signs:

a) A displaced apex beat.
b) Malar flush.
c) A pansystolic murmur best heard at the apex.
d) An early diastolic murmur best heard with the diaphragm of the stethoscope.
e) A mid-diastolic murmur best heard with the bell of the stethoscope.

39. The following are recognized side effects of amiodarone:

a) Hyperthyroidism.
b) Hepatic dysfunction.
c) Xanthopsia.
d) Peripheral neuropathy.
e) Pulmonary fibrosis.

40. The following are characteristic of pericarditis:

a) The chest pain is dull in nature.
b) There may be an associated pericardial effusion.
c) The pericardial rub may come and go.
d) The ECG usually shows regional ST elevation.
e) The ST elevation is concave.

41. The following are features of significant aortic stenosis:

a) Sudden death.
b) An exercise test is contraindicated.
c) The murmur is best heard at the left second intercostal space.
d) The patient may present with angina.
e) The murmur is ejection systolic.

42. Secondary hypertension may be due to the following:

a) Renal artery stenosis.
b) Renal cell carcinoma.
c) Cushing's syndrome.
d) Pregnancy.
e) Oral contraceptive pill.

43. A median sternotomy scar may be used for the following operations:

a) Coronary artery bypass grafting.
b) Aortic valve replacement.
c) Closed mitral valvotomy.
d) Mitral valvuloplasty.
e) Heart transplantation.

44. The following drugs are used in the treatment of hypertension:

a) Atenolol.
b) Doxazocin.
c) Enalapril.
d) Bendrofluazide.
e) Nicorandil.

45. Features of an atrial septal defect include:

a) Fixed splitting of the second heart sound.
b) A harsh machinery murmur heard at the left lower sternal edge.
c) Increased pulmonary blood flow.
d) Possible development of Eisenmenger's syndrome.
e) Central cyanosis from an early age.

46. ECG changes due to myocardial infarction may include the following:

a) ST elevation.
b) Sinus tachycardia.
c) Ventricular tachycardia.
d) Complete heart block.
e) Q waves.

47. The following are contraindications to thrombolysis:

a) Pregnancy.
b) History of haemorrhagic cerebrovascular event more than 6 months previously.
c) Recent gastrointestinal bleed.
d) Warfarin therapy if the international normalized ratio is higher than 1.5.
e) Diabetes mellitus.

48. Complications of myocardial infarction include:

a) Cardiac failure.
b) Mitral regurgitation.
c) Cerebrovascular event.
d) Myocardial rupture.
e) Gastrointestinal bleed.

49. The following drugs have been shown to reduce the mortality rate after myocardial infarction:

a) Streptokinase.
b) Nitrates.
c) Heparin.
d) Aspirin.
e) Angiotensin-converting enzyme inhibitors.

50. The following are effects of chronic excessive alcohol intake:

a) Hypertension.
b) Cardiomyopathy.
c) Sinus bradycardia.
d) Atrial fibrillation.
e) Hypertriglyceridaemia.

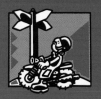

Short-answer Questions

1. List the important steps in the management of a patient who has acute left ventricular failure.

2. Outline the initial investigations in the accident and emergency department you would carry out on a patient who has chest pain. Give the rationale behind each test.

3. Outline the clinical features of syncope that help clarify the underlying cause.

4. Write short notes on the complications of atrial fibrillation.

5. List the peripheral stigmata of infective endocarditis.

6. What does the ECG in Fig. 1 show? Outline the treatment options.

7. Outline the initial investigations in the accident and emergency department of a patient who has suspected infective endocarditis.

8. What does the ECG in Fig. 2 show? List two possible underlying causes.

9. Write short notes on the complications of cardiac catheterization.

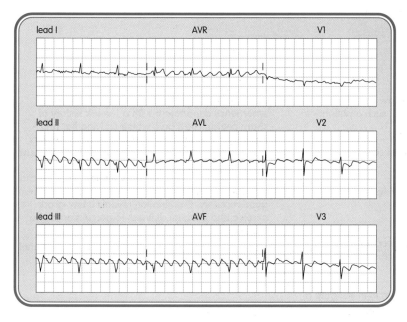

Fig. 1

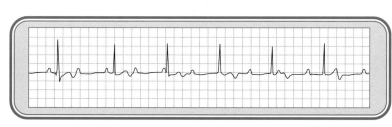

Fig. 2

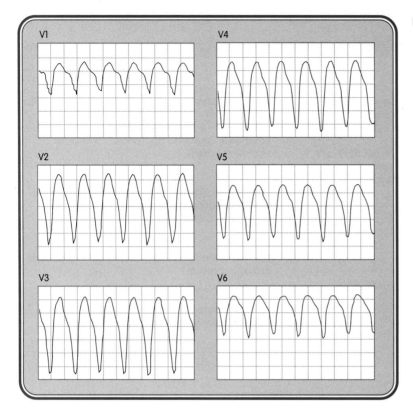

Fig. 3

V1

V4

V2

V5

V3

V6

10. What does Fig. 3. show? Draw a flow chart to describe the acute management of such a patient.

11. Describe the physical signs of mitral stenosis.

12. What diagnosis is shown by Fig. 4? Approximately how long ago did this happen?

13. What are the clinical findings you would expect to see in a child who has a patent ductus arteriosus?

14. Which blood tests would you request to investigate a patient who has ankle oedema and why?

15. A 60-year-old man presents to the accident and emergency department with a 1-week history of sharp central chest pain worse on lying flat and inspiration and relieved by sitting forward. He has also noticed increasing breathlessness over the past 48 hours and some discomfort in both knees. Of note in his past medical history he had a myocardial infarction 6 weeks previously from which he made a good recovery. Examination reveals a low-grade pyrexia and bilateral dullness to percussion at the lung bases.

a) What is the most likely diagnosis and why?
b) What are your main differential diagnoses?

Fig. 4

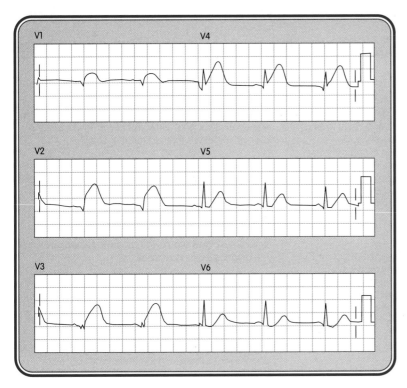

V1   V4

V2   V5

V3   V6

16. A 40-year-old publican presents to the accident and emergency department with a 4-month history of gradually increasing shortness of breath. This breathlessness is worse on exertion and on lying flat and he now needs to use four pillows at night to prop himself up. Over the past 2 weeks he has noticed that his legs are swollen, especially at the end of each day. He denies any chest pain or palpitations. The social history reveals that he has smoked 20 cigarettes a day from the age of 16 years and that he drinks approximately 60 units of alcohol each week. He has no family history of heart disease.

a) What diagnosis do the symptoms suggest?
b) What is the most likely cause ?
c) Give two possible differential diagnoses?

17. Write short notes on streptokinase.

18. List the possible complications that may be seen within the first 7 days after a myocardial infarction.

19. Give four possible indications for implantation of a permanent pacemaker.

20. A young woman attends the outpatient clinic. She has a confirmed diagnosis of atrial septal defect and she is currently well. She has been told she needs antibiotic prophylaxis before certain procedures, but is unsure which ones, how would you advise her?

Patient Management Problems

1. A 65-year-old man presents with a 3-hour history of central crushing chest pain radiating down the left arm. Of note he is a smoker of many years and his brother has had a coronary artery bypass operation. On examination he is sweaty and anxious. Blood pressure is 150/90 mmHg and the examination is otherwise normal. Initial ECG shows ST segment elevation of 2 mm in leads V4–V6, I, and AVL. Describe the management of this patient during the first few hours of his admission.

2. The man described in Patient Management Problem 1 above has recovered well and is ready for discharge from hospital 1 week later. He is seen as an outpatient 2 months later and complains of central chest pain on exertion that is relieved by rest. What medication would he have been discharged on and why? How would you investigate his current chest pain?

3. A 50-year-old lorry driver is admitted with a history of sudden tearing chest pain radiating between the shoulder blades. He has a history of hypertension and has been a smoker for many years. On examination he is sweaty with a blood pressure of 120/80 mmHg in the right arm and 90/60 mmHg in the left. He has a tachycardia and on auscultation there is a murmur of aortic regurgitation. What is the most likely diagnosis? What initial investigations would you carry out urgently? Outline the management of this condition.

4. As a junior doctor you are asked to speak to a group of young people about prevention of ischaemic heart disease. What would you say?

5. A 60-year-old woman is seen in outpatients with a history of recurrent collapse. She describes the episodes as having no precipitating events and occurring with no warning. She loses consciousness for a few seconds and feels relatively well on regaining consciousness. She is on no medication and has no past medical history of note. The episodes have recently begun to occur more frequently and she is currently experiencing them approximately once every week. Examination is entirely unremarkable. What is the most likely cause for the episodes? What are the differential diagnoses? What investigations would you perform to find the cause of the collapses.

6. A 70-year-old woman is seen by you with a suspected diagnosis of aortic stenosis. What would you expect to see on examination? How would you investigate this patient? What are the treatment options?

7. A 20-year-old intravenous drug abuser presents to the accident and emergency department with fever, rash, and a pansystolic murmur. You suspect infective endocarditis. What are the differential diagnoses for the pansystolic murmur? What are the likely causative organisms? How would you manage this patient once the diagnosis was confirmed.

8. A 40-year-old man presents with evidence of a pericardial effusion on echocardiogram. The pericardial fluid is tapped and turns out to be an effusion. What signs would you expect to find on examination if there was cardiac tamponade? What is an effusion? What could the underlying cause be?

9. A 48-year-old investment banker has presented to the outpatient clinic with newly diagnosed hypertension. He is keen to know about the possible drugs used in the treatment of hypertension and their side effects. Briefly outline the possible agents and their more common side effects.

10. A 56-year-old man who has a positive coronary angiogram is found to have a random cholesterol level of 7.5 mmol/L. What physical signs may be found on examination that suggest this result? What further investigatons would be appropriate? Should he be treated? Why? How would you manage his hypercholesterolaemia?

1.	a)T,	b)T,	c)T,	d)F,	e)F
2.	a)T,	b)T,	c)T,	d)F	e)T
3.	a)F,	b)T,	c)T,	d)F,	e)T
4.	a)T,	b)T,	c)T,	d)T,	e)T
5.	a)T,	b)T,	c)F,	d)T,	e)F
6.	a)T,	b)T,	c)T,	d)T,	e)T
7.	a)T,	b)T,	c)T,	d)T,	e)T
8.	a)T,	b)F,	c)F,	d)T,	e)T
9.	a)F,	b)T,	c)T,	d)T,	e)T
10.	a)F,	b)F,	c)T,	d)F,	e)F
11.	a)T,	b)T,	c)T,	d)F,	e)T
12.	a)T,	b)F,	c)T,	d)F,	e)F
13.	a)T,	b)T,	c)T,	d)T,	e)F
14.	a)T,	b)T,	c)T	d)F,	e)T
15.	a)T,	b)T,	c)F,	d)T,	e)T
16.	a)T,	b)T,	c)T,	d)T,	e)F
17.	a)T,	b)T,	c)T,	d)F,	e)T
18.	a)F,	b)T,	c)T,	d)T,	e)T
19.	a)F,	b)T,	c)T,	d)T,	e)F
20.	a)T,	b)T,	c)T,	d)T,	e)F
21.	a)T,	b)T,	c)T,	d)F,	e)F
22.	a)T,	b)T,	c)T,	d)F,	e)F
23.	a)T,	b)F,	c)F,	d)F,	e)T
24.	a)T,	b)F,	c)T,	d)T,	e)F
25.	a)T,	b)T,	c)T,	d)F,	e)F
26.	a)T,	b)T,	c)T,	d)T,	e)F
27.	a)F,	b)T,	c)T,	d)F,	e)T
28.	a)F,	b)T,	c)F,	d)T,	e)T
29.	a)F,	b)F,	c)T,	d)F,	e)T
30.	a)F,	b)T,	c)F,	d)F,	e)F
31.	a)F,	b)T,	c)T,	d)F,	e)T
32.	a)T,	b)T,	c)F,	d)T,	e)T
33.	a)F,	b)T,	c)T,	d)F,	e)F
34.	a)F,	b)F,	c)F,	d)F,	e)T
35.	a)T,	b)T,	c)F,	d)T,	e)T
36.	a)T,	b)T,	c)F,	d)T,	e)T
37.	a)F,	b)T,	c)T,	d)T,	e)T
38.	a)F,	b)T,	c)F,	d)F,	e)T
39.	a)T,	b)T,	c)F,	d)T,	e)T
40.	a)F,	b)T,	c)T,	d)F,	e)T
41.	a)T,	b)T,	c)F,	d)T,	e)T
42.	a)T,	b)F,	c)T,	d)T,	e)T
43.	a)T,	b)T,	c)F,	d)F,	e)T
44.	a)T,	b)T,	c)T,	d)T,	e)F
45.	a)T,	b)F,	c)T,	d)T,	e)F
46.	a)T,	b)T,	c)T,	d)T,	e)T
47.	a)T,	b)T,	c)T,	d)T,	e)F
48.	a)T,	b)T,	c)T,	d)T,	e)F
49.	a)T,	b)F,	c)F,	d)T,	e)T
50.	a)T,	b)T,	c)F,	d)T,	e)T

1. • Sit the patient up.
   • Administer oxygen (100%) via a facial mask.
   • Establish intravenous access and administer the following: diamorphine 2.5–5 mg; metoclopramide 10 mg; frusemide 80 mg.
   • Insert a urethral catheter.
   • Consider the need for intravenous nitrate infusion.
   • Continue to monitor the patient with regular measurements of blood pressure and blood oxygen saturation.

2. • A full blood count—to exclude anaemia, which can precipitate angina. A patient who has pneumonia or a myocardial infarction may have a leucocytosis.
   • Urea and electrolytes—to show any renal impairment that may affect subsequent drug therapy or may worsen if the patient is hypotensive. Hypokalaemia is an important cause of arrhythmias in patients after myocardial infarction.
   • Liver function tests and amylase—may be abnormal if the chest pain is due to cholecystitis or pancreatitis.
   • Cardiac enzymes—if elevated suggest acute myocardial infarction.
   • Electrocardiogram—this may show ST segment depression in angina or regional ST elevation in myocardial infarction. Global ST elevation that is saddle shaped suggests pericarditis. If large a pulmonary embolus may result in the classical S1,Q3,T3 appearance.
   • Chest radiograph—may show pulmonary oedema in a patient who has a myocardial infarction. Pulmonary embolus may produce a region of oligaemia on the chest film. Widening of the mediastinum suggests aortic dissection.

3. • The precipitating factors—may point to a cause (e.g. painful stimuli suggests a vasovagal cause).
   • Speed of onset is important—sudden onset suggests a cardiac or cerebrovascular cause whereas gradual onset suggests a metabolic cause.
   • Presence or absence of warning signs—cardiac syncope usually occurs without warning whereas epilepsy or hypoglycaemia are usually preceded by specific symptoms.
   • Witness account of the period of unconsciousness—specifically the presence of tonic–clonic movements, tongue biting, or incontinence, all of which suggest epileptiform seizures
   • Speed and nature of recovery—cardiac syncope is usually followed by a rapid recovery but a patient will often be very drowsy after an epileptic seizure.

4. • Complications secondary to persistent tachycardia, which may lead to cardiac failure. Angina may also be exacerbated by the tachycardia.
   • Complications secondary to thromboembolism. The stasis of blood within the atria may lead to intracardiac clot formation and subsequent embolization may manifest as stroke, mesenteric infarction, or infarction of the fingers or toes.

5. • Hands—splinter haemorrhages, clubbing, Osler's nodes Janeway lesions.
   • Skin—vasculitic rash.
   • Urine—microscopic haematuria.
   • Eyes—Roth's spots, conjunctival haemorrhages.
   • Neurological system, focal neurological defect.
   • Peripheral infarcts.
   • Joints—arthritis and swelling.

6. • Atrial flutter with slow ventricular response (4 to 1 block).
   • Treatment options include DC cardioversion with a synchronized shock—the patient should be fully anticoagulated with warfarin because there is a risk of thromboembolism. Cardioversion using drug therapy could be attempted using class III antiarrhythmic agents such as sotalol or amiodarone, but these may slow the ventricular rate further, resulting in hypotension secondary to profound bradycardia.
   • As the ventricular rate is already slow rate control using class II or IV agents is not indicated.
   • In all cases the underlying cause for the atrial flutter should be sought and treated.

7. • Blood tests—three sets of blood cultures should be performed at least 1 hour apart before antibiotics are started if the patient is well enough. A full blood count is performed to look for a leucocytosis and for anaemia of chronic disease. Urea and electrolytes will exclude renal failure, which may be a consequence of endocarditis and may influence the drug therapy. Liver function may be deranged in sepsis.
   • Chest radiograph—this may show evidence of left ventricular failure.
   • Electrocardiogram—there may be a sinus tachycardia. Heart block is an extremely serious sign and suggests the presence of a septal abscess.

8. • Complete heart block.
   • Possible causes include inferior myocardial infarction, drug therapy (especially with antiarrhythmic agents), congenital complete heart block, septal abscess, aortic valve replacement.

9.
- Complications involving the puncture site include haemorrhage, excessive bruising, and pseudoaneurysm formation, The puncture site may become infected.
- The artery used for access may become thrombosed resulting in an ischaemic leg or arm.
- Trauma caused by the catheter may result in embolization of pieces of plaque to the cardiac, cerebral, or peripheral circulation causing myocardial infarction, cerebrovascular event, ischaemic toes or hands, or mesenteric infarcts.
- Myocardial or coronary artery tears may occur resulting in haemopericardium and possibly pericardial tamponade.
- Anaphylactic reactions to the dye used may occur and in some cases are fatal.

10.
- The patient has developed ventricular tachycardia.
- See Fig. 5. It is very important that you know the algorithms for basic and advanced life support (see also Figs 17.1 & 17.4).

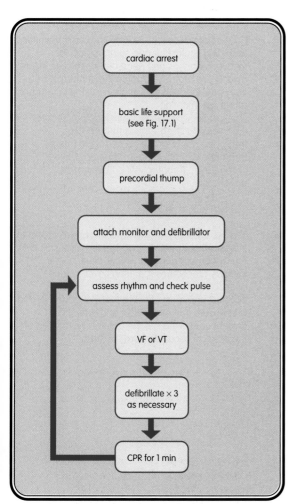

Fig. 5

11.
- The patient may be dyspnoeic.
- The patient may have a malar flush.
- The patient may be in atrial fibrillation so the pulse is irregularly irregular.
- The apex beat is not displaced and is tapping in nature.
- There may be a loud first heart sound.
- There is an opening snap after the second heart sound followed by a low rumbling mid-diastolic murmur heard best at the apex with the patient lying on his or her left side and in full expiration.
- If pulmonary hypertension has developed there is a loud pulmonary component of the second heart sound (P_2) and a left parasternal heave.
- If the pulmonary hypertension has led to right ventricular impairment the jugular venous pressure will be elevated and there will be peripheral oedema, ascites, and hepatomegaly. There may be tricuspid regurgitation.

12.
- Anteroseptal myocardial infarction.
- There are no Q waves therefore the onset must have been less than 24 hours previously.

13.
- A patent ductus arteriosus occurs if there is failure of the closure of the fetal connection between the pulmonary artery and the aorta after birth. Blood therefore passes from the high pressure aorta into the lower pressure pulmonary system, creating a left-to-right shunt.
- If the shunt is large the child may be breathless due to left ventricular failure, and there is failure to thrive, so the child may be small and underweight.
- On examination the pulse is collapsing in nature and of high volume.
- The cardiac apex is thrusting and may be displaced downward and laterally if there is left ventricular failure. There is a palpable thrill at the second left intercostal space. On auscultation at the same place there is a loud continuous machinery murmur obscuring the second heart sound.
- If the shunt is large and pulmonary hypertension develops there may be reversal of the shunt and Eisenmenger's syndrome occurs—this causes differential cyanosis (cyanosed feet and pink hands) and usually develops after several years so is unlikely to be seen in a young child.

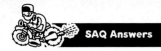

14. • Full blood count—anaemia can precipitate cardiac failure and is also seen in other disease (e.g. renal impairment, hypothyroidism).
    • Renal function (urea and electrolytes)—renal impairment may cause ankle oedema. Patients who have longstanding cardiac or hepatic impairment often have deranged renal function.
    • Liver function tests—deranged in hepatic failure.
    • Plasma albumin concentration—reduced in protein-losing states such as nephrotic syndrome or protein-losing gastroenteropathy, but also reduced in any chronic disease state.
    • Thyroid function tests—hyperthyroidism may precipitate cardiac failure.
    • In addition to these baseline tests it may be appropriate to exclude Cushing's disease by performing cortisol measurements and a dexamethasone suppression test.

15. a) The pain described is classically pericarditic and in a patient 6 weeks after a myocardial infarction suspect Dressler's syndrome as being the diagnosis. Dressler's syndrome is also associated with pleurisy (which would explain the bilateral pleural effusions) and arthritis.
    b) The main differential diagnoses would be:
    • Pericarditis of another cause (e.g. viral causes such as coxsackievirus and enterovirus).
    • Pulmonary embolus—must be considered in any patient who is breathless after an illness.
    • Pneumonia—especially if the organism is atypical (e.g. mycoplasma)—may also cause chest pain on breathing, pleural effusions, arthralgia, and a low-grade fever.

16. a) The symptoms suggest a diagnosis of congestive cardiac failure—suggested by dyspnoea, orthopnoea and oedema.
    b) The most likely cause is chronic heavy alcohol consumption resulting in alcoholic cardiomyopathy.
    c) Other possible causes are ischaemic heart disease and haemochromatosis.

17. • Streptokinase is a protein derived from β-haemolytic streptococci.
    • It has been shown to reduce the mortality rate in patients who have acute myocardial infarction when given within 24 hours of the onset of pain.
    • Streptokinase acts by binding to plasminogen to form a complex that activates to convert another molecule of plasminogen to plasmin. This results in fibrinolysis and breakdown of thrombus. Streptokinase acts on all plasminogen—it is not clot specific.
    • The drug is given as a 1-hour long intravenous infusion of 1.5 million units.
    • It has a half life of 18 min, but the complex with plasminogen has a half-life of 180 min.
    • Side effects and complications of streptokinase include anaphylaxis, hypotension, and haemorrhage.
    • Antibody production to the drug renders subsequent doses less effective, therefore many centres will not use streptokinase more than once in the same patient.

18. • Cardiac complications include cardiac arrhythmias (including ventricular and supraventricular tachyarrhythmias and heart block), cardiac failure, myocardial rupture including the septum or free wall, papillary muscle rupture resulting in torrential mitral regurgitation.
    • Non-cardiac complications include pulmonary embolus and deep venous thrombosis, thromboembolic stroke secondary to mural thrombus formation, haemorrhagic stroke secondary to thrombolysis adminstration, pneumonia.

19. • See Fig. 18.9, p. 143.

20. • See Fig. 23.3, p. 178. The most important aspect to stress is that any dental work, even a session with the hygienist requires antibiotic cover. Other invasive procedures requiring cover include operations of any sort and cystoscopy. The simplest and most effective piece of advice to give is to ensure that all medical and dental professionals who see the patient are advised of the medical condition from the start.

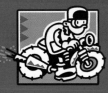

Index

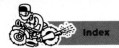

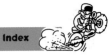